# Enamel and Dentin-Pulp Complex

*Edited by Lavinia Cosmina Ardelean and Laura-Cristina Rusu*

Published in London, United Kingdom

Enamel and Dentin-Pulp Complex
http://dx.doi.org/10.5772/intechopen.114766
Edited by Lavinia Cosmina Ardelean and Laura-Cristina Rusu

Contributors
Abubaker El Elhaj, Alexandra Roi, Atena Galuscan, Codruța Victoria Țigmeanu, Cristian Danilo Urgiles, Cristina Estefania Urgiles Esquivel, Daniela Jumanca, Daniela San Martin, Darren Dhananthat Chawhuaveang, Divya Mudumba, Fernanda Gonzalez, Kusumawadee Utispan, Laura-Cristina Rusu, Lavinia Cosmina Ardelean, María Isabel Bravo, Merita Barani-Sveçla, Ollie Yiru Yu, Ramona Dumitrescu, Rattapong Worawongvasu, Shqipe Buleshkaj, Sittichai Koontongkaew



First published in London, United Kingdom, 2024 by IntechOpen
IntechOpen is the global imprint of INTECHOPEN LIMITED, registered in England and Wales, registration number: 11086078, 167-169 Great Portland Street, London, W1W 5PF, United Kingdom

British Library Cataloguing-in-Publication Data
A catalogue record for this book is available from the British Library

Additional hard and PDF copies can be obtained from orders@intechopen.com

Enamel and Dentin-Pulp Complex
Edited by Lavinia Cosmina Ardelean and Laura-Cristina Rusu
p. cm.

This title is part of the Dentistry Book Series, Volume 18
Topic: Oral Health
Series Editor: Sergio Alexandre Gehrke
Topic Editor: Sandra Marinho and Esra Guzeldemir-Akcakanat

Print ISBN 978-0-85014-015-6
Online ISBN 978-0-85014-016-3
eBook (PDF) ISBN 978-0-85014-017-0
ISSN 2631-6218

For EU product safety concerns:
IN TECH d.o.o., Prolaz Marije Krucifikse Kozulić 3, 51000 Rijeka, Croatia,
info@intechopen.com or visit our website at intechopen.com.

IntechOpen Book Series

# Dentistry

Volume 18

## Aims and Scope of the Series

This book series will offer a comprehensive overview of recent research trends as well as clinical applications within different specialties of dentistry. Topics will include overviews of the health of the oral cavity, from prevention and care to different treatments for the rehabilitation of problems that may affect the organs and/or tissues present. The different areas of dentistry will be explored, with the aim of disseminating knowledge and providing readers with new tools for the comprehensive treatment of their patients with greater safety and with current techniques. Ongoing issues, recent advances, and future diagnostic approaches and therapeutic strategies will also be discussed. This series of books will focus on various aspects of the properties and results obtained by the various treatments available, whether preventive or curative.

# Meet the Series Editor

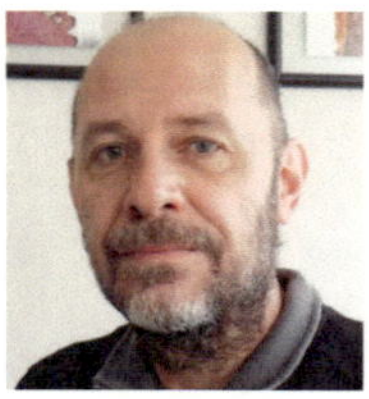

Dr. Sergio Alexandre Gehrke is a doctorate holder in two fields. The first is a Ph.D. in Cellular and Molecular Biology from the Pontificia Catholic University, Porto Alegre, Brazil, in 2010 and the other is an International Ph.D. in Bioengineering from the Universidad Miguel Hernandez, Elche/Alicante, Spain, obtained in 2020. In 2018, he completed a postdoctoral fellowship in Materials Engineering in the NUCLEMAT of the Pontificia Catholic University, Porto Alegre, Brazil. He is currently the Director of the Postgraduate Program in Implantology of the Bioface/UCAM/PgO (Montevideo, Uruguay), Director of the Cathedra of Biotechnology of the Catholic University of Murcia (Murcia, Spain), an Extraordinary Full Professor of the Catholic University of Murcia (Murcia, Spain) as well as the Director of the private center of research Biotecnos – Technology and Science (Montevideo, Uruguay). Applied biomaterials, cellular and molecular biology, and dental implants are among his research interests. He has published several original papers in renowned journals. In addition, he is also a Collaborating Professor in several Postgraduate programs at different universities all over the world.

# Meet the Volume Editors

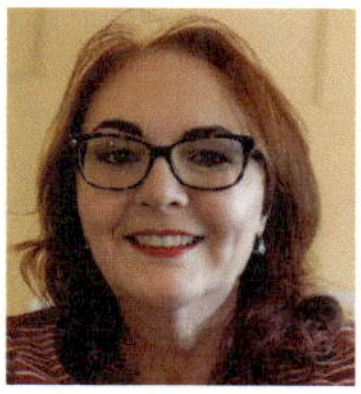

Professor Lavinia Cosmina Ardelean, DMD, Ph.D., is a professor and head of the Department of Technology of Materials and Devices in Dental Medicine, "Victor Babes" University of Medicine and Pharmacy, Timisoara, Romania. She has authored/co-authored 19 books, 15 book chapters, and more than 120 peer-reviewed papers. She is an editorial board member of numerous journals and a member of reviewer/topic boards of the journals *Materials*, *Prosthesis*, *Metals*, *Coatngs*, *Polymers*, and *Journal of Functonal Biomaterials*. She has served as guest editor for ten special journal issues and six books. Being an actve reviewer, with more than 270 reviews to her credit to date, Dr. Ardelean was awarded the Top Reviewers in Cross-Field Award and Top Reviewers in Materials Science Award in 2019. She currently holds two patents. Her research interest includes most areas of dentstry, with a focus on dental materials/biomaterials, dental alloys, resins, ceramics/bioceramics, CAD/CAM milling, 3D printng/bioprintng in dentstry, welding, scanning, prosthodontcs, and oral health care.

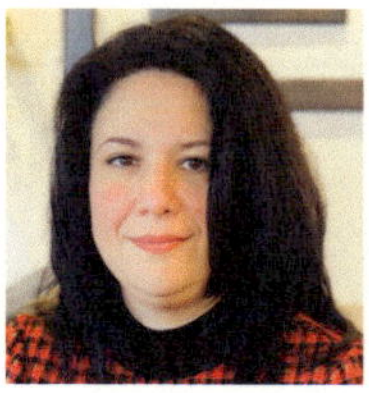

Professor Laura Cristna Rusu, DMD, Ph.D., is the mother of two lovely boys and a full-tme professor and head of the Oral Pathology Department, Faculty of Dental Medicine, "Victor Babes" University of Medicine and Pharmacy, Timisoara, Romania. Her Ph.D. thesis was centered on allergens in dental materials. In 2017 she obtained a Dr Habil and was confrmed as Ph.D. coordinator in the feld of dental medicine. She took part in 11 research projects, including FP7 COST Acton MP 1005, and authored more than 140 peer-reviewed papers. She has published ten books and book chapters as author and co-author. She has guest-edited seven special issues in diferent journals and edited or co-edited fve books, plus one ongoing book editng project. She currently holds three patents. Dr. Rusu is a member of the editorial board of *Journal of Science and Art* and *Medicine in Evoluton*, and a topic editor for the journal *Materials*. Her main scientfc interests are oral pathology and oral diagnosis in dental medicine, focusing on oral cancer.

# Contents

# Preface

Enamel is a unique component of tooth structure, mainly due to its high mineral content and protective role for the inner, more fragile dentin-pulp complex, being the first and most important line of defense against tooth decay.

The dentin and pulp are embryologically, histologically, and functionally similar tissues, being considered complex. The dentin-pulp complex consists of an outer hard tissue layer, the dentin, and the inner soft tissue layer, the vital pulp, with its network of nerves, vascular, and fibrous elements. The dentin-pulp complex has an essential role in maintaining a functional viable tooth by supporting the enamel in dissipating the masticatory forces as well as maintaining tissue homeostasis.

During the developmental process, the enamel and dentin structure may be affected by genetic and environmental factors, which may result in defects that impair their biology and function.

A deep knowledge and understanding of sound and affected tooth structures enables proper diagnosis and pertinent treatment options.

Maintaining proper tooth function is an important factor in ensuring a high quality of life. However, improper hygiene, illness, injury, and aging may result in impaired tooth function, which requires appropriate restoral approaches.

Being the external protective layer of the tooth, enamel preservation should be a priority. This can be accomplished by following a proper diet and dental routine and implementing early preventive treatment. When the enamel is damaged, hypersensitivity and caries are likely to occur.

Left untreated, caries will progress and cause damage to the dentin-pulp complex, ultimately destroying the crown, perforating the pulp cavity, and causing pulp inflammation and pain.

The goal of modern society, from the perspective of oral health, consists of prevention, proper diagnosis, better dental care, and novel treatment options. The aim of developing new appropriate methods for restoring tooth function not only results in a wide range of materials, including smart ones, and computerized technologies, but also in implementing tissue engineering in the dental field.

Tissue engineering provides an attractive option to regenerate and replace dental tissues and even to obtain a full tooth structure. It requires the integration of key elements such as stem cells, extracellular matrix scaffold, and growth factor. The dental pulp is an important source of stem cells, which can proliferate and differentiate, thus contributing to treating various health issues or playing a crucial role in tissue regeneration, for both oral and non-oral areas. Pulp stem cells are, therefore, a promising source for a variety of clinical applications.

This book, consisting of seven chapters, focuses on important aspects of preventing and treating dental caries, as well as novel materials and regeneration issues.

**Lavinia Cosmina Ardelean**
Department of Technology of Materials and Devices in Dental Medicine,
Multidisciplinary Center for Research, Evaluation, Diagnosis
and Therapies in Oral Medicine,
"Victor Babeș" University of Medicine and Pharmacy Timisoara,
Timisoara, Romania

**Laura-Cristina Rusu**
Department of Oral Pathology,
Multidisciplinary Center for Research, Evaluation, Diagnosis
and Therapies in Oral Medicine,
"Victor Babeș" University of Medicine and Pharmacy Timisoara,
Timisoara, Romania

Chapter 1

# Etiopathogenesis of Dental Caries

*Merita Barani-Sveçla and Shqipe Buleshkaj*

## Abstract

Dental caries, as a pervasive and complex global health issue affecting individuals of all ages, is influenced by a multitude of factors. These factors encompass the interplay of demineralization and remineralization processes, dietary and oral hygiene practices, salivary composition and flow, tooth morphology, genetics, fluoride exposure, and environmental and socioeconomic variables. This chapter analyzes three categories of factors that cause dental caries, such as: general, local, and iatrogenic factors. Initially, the genetic predisposition, gender-related hormonal fluctuations, aging, immunological elements, pregnancy-related changes, chronic diseases, hormonal disorders, vitamin levels, and socioeconomic factors are included in general factors that contribute to the susceptibility to dental caries. Moreover, to understand and mitigate caries risk, it is pivotal to analyze local factors such as dental morphology, oral hygiene, and the vital role of saliva. Additionally, premature loss of primary teeth, crowding, orthodontic treatment, dental fillings, and prosthetic dental work can lead to iatrogenic issues affecting oral health. Recognizing the multifaceted nature of dental caries, susceptibility underscores the necessity for comprehensive strategies in oral health care. Therefore, this chapter underlines that proper oral care, preventive measures, and meticulous attention during dental procedures are paramount for maintaining optimal oral health.

**Keywords:** dental caries, general factors, local factors, iatrogenic factors, oral health care

## 1. Introduction

Tooth decay, commonly known as dental caries, is a widespread chronic disease affecting people of all ages and demographics. Often seen as just a minor discomfort, it significantly impacts not only dental health but also overall well-being and quality of life [1]. Dental caries arises from a complex mix of genetic, environmental, behavioral, and iatrogenic factors, illustrating its multifaceted origins.

The development and progression of dental caries are influenced by various factors, which this chapter categorizes into general, local, and iatrogenic. General factors include heredity, gender, age, immunological factors, hormones, vitamins, and diet, each playing a unique role in an individual's vulnerability to tooth decay [2–4]. These elements underscore the importance of understanding the interaction between internal physiological processes and external environmental conditions. Factors like genetic predispositions, hormonal changes, and dietary choices work together, influencing both the risk and the actual development of dental caries [5, 6].

Local factors, such as dental morphology, oral hygiene, and saliva, are also crucial in caries development, highlighting the significance of physical characteristics and personal habits. The structure and alignment of teeth and the composition and flow of saliva greatly affect the likelihood of developing caries [7, 8]. Additionally, iatrogenic factors, which are unintended consequences of medical or dental treatments, can also contribute to the development of caries [9].

This chapter aims to offer a comprehensive perspective on the various factors influencing dental caries, enhancing understanding of the complexities in its prevention and management. It emphasizes the need for personalized dental care approaches, tailored to each individual's unique risk factors and dental characteristics [10]. The chapter also acknowledges the ongoing need for research and innovation in dental science to develop more effective strategies for preventing and treating dental caries.

Addressing dental caries effectively requires a thorough understanding of its etiology and a comprehensive approach to intervention. This overview aims to provide dental professionals with fundamental insights for designing effective, personalized prevention and treatment strategies. We explore the diverse aspects of dental caries as we delve into the complexities of this common yet intricate condition.

In summary, we examine the most important factors of tooth decay. A.D.A. (American Dental Association) makes the classification of direct and indirect factors of caries presentation. Our classification will be according to F.D.I. (International Dental Federation), according to which the division is made into three categories thoroughly presented and described in this chapter:

The research methodology applied in this chapter, which primarily relies on a literature review, is the systematic review [11] and meta-analysis [12] approach. This methodology is particularly suited for synthesizing a wide range of research findings from various studies to provide a comprehensive understanding of a complex subject like dental caries. This systematic review and meta-analysis approach provides a structured and comprehensive way to analyze the existing literature on dental caries, ensuring that the conclusions drawn are based on a thorough and unbiased evaluation of current research.

## 2. General factors

Six general factors are presented in this chapter including: heredity, gender, age, imunological factor, hormones, and vitamins and food.

### 2.1 Heredity

By heredity we mean that one family has a predisposition for the appearance of caries compared to the other. In contrast to it, there are families where the caries percentage coefficient is much smaller, which is justified by genetic factors [13].

Genes play a role in dental caries development, but the condition's origin is influenced by a complex interplay of environmental and genetic factors. To validate these findings across diverse populations, further research is needed. Identifying genetic risk factors is essential for screening susceptible individuals and deepening our understanding of gene involvement in caries development. Insights from these studies offer valuable tools for efficiently implementing advanced preventive measures, diagnostics, and innovative therapies in managing the disease [14].

Differences in the oral microbiome arise from a combination of genetic and peripheral factors. In the symbiotic relationship between microorganisms and the host, homeostasis in the oral microbiome is typically maintained. However, certain conditions may shift this balance toward a parasitic relationship, leading to the proliferation of cariogenic microorganisms and the development of dental caries. Advanced molecular biology techniques have enabled the discovery of new species of cariogenic microorganisms. It's important to note that each person's oral microbiome is unique, making commonly adopted disease prevention measures not universally applicable to all individuals [15].

Host genetics stands out as a pivotal factor contributing to variations in susceptibility to caries among individuals. Numerous genes influence an individual's likelihood of developing caries by playing crucial roles in immune response, saliva production, and tooth enamel development. On a global scale, scientists are engaged in genetic studies to explore various diseases, including dental caries [16, 17]. Experimental studies have revealed a genetic impact on caries outcomes, distinguishing between susceptible and resistant strains [18].

Studies indicate that specific genes influence enamel resistance, while another set affects salivary composition and the host's response to infection. Furthermore, numerous linkages and association studies have identified genomic regions and polymorphisms associated with dental caries. This extensive research underscores the multifaceted genetic factors contributing to variations in caries susceptibility [14, 19, 20].

Caries risk and resistance are influenced by a multitude of genetic factors encompassing taste preference, salivary attributes, immune response, tooth morphology, enamel composition and structure, and behavioral traits. Unlike Mendelian inheritance, where a single gene may have a major effect, dental caries, being a chronic and complex disease, is likely influenced by the interplay of multiple genes. Additionally, gene-gene interactions or gene-environment interactions may give rise to epigenetic effects, further contributing to the intricate balance between risk and resistance associated with dental caries. The holistic understanding of these diverse genetic factors highlights the complexity of the genetic landscape influencing susceptibility to and protection against dental caries [7, 8].

### 2.2 Gender

Gender inequalities in dental health, particularly in terms of caries and periodontal diseases among adults, have been extensively studied [21–23]. Numerous findings indicate that women tend to experience a higher burden of dental caries, possibly due to hormonal changes leading to increased viscosity and reduced saliva production. The average pH of women's saliva is lower than that of men, 7.2 and 7.5, respectively [13]. Studies consistently show that females, across different age groups, are at a higher risk of and experience more carious lesions than males. Several factors contribute to this discrepancy, such as earlier tooth eruption in girls, variations in dietary behaviors, access to oral health care, hormonal differences, and characteristics of dentition, tooth enamel, or saliva.

Additionally, gender may influence oral health habits, with men often neglecting their oral health and displaying poorer habits. Research indicates that women generally perceive oral health as having a greater impact on quality of life, associating poor oral health with pain and embarrassment. Furthermore, studies reveal that women tend to have better oral health literacy and more positive attitudes toward dental visits compared to men [24–29].

## 2.3 Age

Tooth decay is more a disease of young people. Some periods of life are distinguished by a higher index of caries appearance.

The age of 5 to 8 years is characterized by a higher percentage of caries, and then it rapidly declines with the eruption of permanent teeth. The period of adolescence (13–20 years old) is again considered as a period with more caries, which is followed by stabilization until the age of 40–50 years, where caries is combined with periodontopathy [13].

Aging is a natural physiological process characterized by changes over time, occurring at varying rates influenced by lifestyle, environment, and genetics. Distinguishing between normal aging and disease can be challenging. In the oral cavity, aging is marked by enamel wear, chipping, fracture lines, and a darker tooth color. Deposition of secondary dentin reduces the size of pulp chambers and canals. Coronal or root caries, however, signifies disease.

Limited periodontal attachment loss is associated with aging, often seen as recession on the buccal surface. Severe periodontitis peaks at 35–40 years, affecting 10.5–12% of the population. Mucosal tissue changes with age, including reduced wound-healing capacity. Smoking significantly increases the risk of mucosal pathology. Reduced salivary gland function is linked to medication usage and disorders like diabetes, more prevalent in older adults [30].

Masticatory function is crucial for older adults, promoting a nutritionally complete diet to prevent sarcopenia and frailty syndrome. Successful oral aging is defined by adequate function and comfort, with a proposal for 20 functional teeth in occlusion as a measure. Healthy oral aging contributes to overall healthy aging, encompassing both biological and social well-being.

## 2.4 Imunological factor

The likelihood of developing tooth decay in individuals is influenced by various factors, including the immune system and the oral microbiome. The oral microbiome, in turn, is shaped by both environmental and genetic determinants. These interrelated elements contribute to the complex dynamics of oral health, highlighting the importance of understanding how genetic and environmental factors interact to impact an individual's susceptibility to tooth decay [15].

Recent research shows that the appearance of caries is directly dependent on the presence of secretory immunoglobulin IgA in saliva. The amount of IgA less than 14.2 mg/100 ml in saliva enables the rapid development of Streptococus mutans, one of the most dangerous causes for the appearance of caries [13].

Antibodies against oral bacteria, including Streptococus mutans, can be identified in both human serum and saliva. Numerous studies comparing caries experience and the levels of immunoglobulin or specific antibodies have been conducted to explore the potential role of these antibodies in natural caries immunity. However, a consistent pattern in the results of such experiments is not evident. Several small-scale human trials in adults have demonstrated the feasibility of elevating levels of salivary S-IgA antibodies against Streptococus mutans. In some instances, these antibodies were shown to interfere with the colonization of Streptococus mutans [31].

Chronic diseases - patients suffering from chronic diseases have a higher prevalence of caries. Patients with myocardial infarction, diabetes mellitus, or duodenal ulcer present differently in the oral cavity due to medications, ketonic bodies (change in the pH of saliva), and fetor ex ore. All these are predisposing factors for the development of microorganisms and the greater appearance of caries [13].

Poor oral health is associated with an increased likelihood of developing respiratory and cardiovascular diseases, adverse pregnancy outcomes, and diabetes mellitus. The role of oral microorganisms in the etiology and progression of these conditions is becoming increasingly recognized. Current knowledge on oral dysbiosis sheds light on the pathophysiologic mechanisms involving oral microorganisms in each of these health issues [32].

Within oral pathology, various diseases such as dental caries, periodontal diseases, endodontic infections, and even oral cancer have been linked to oral microorganisms. Beyond oral health, systemic diseases like nonoral infections, adverse pregnancy outcomes, cardiovascular diseases, and diabetes are prevalent pathologies with established connections to microorganisms in the oral cavity. Understanding these associations is crucial for comprehensive healthcare management and preventive measures [33].

### 2.5 Hormones and vitamins

Any hormone disorder manifested in the form of hyperfunction or hypofunction of the thymus, pituitary, thyroid, and parathyroid as a consequence causes the appearance of caries in a larger percentage [13].

The oral health needs of women and men exhibit significant differences, with hormonal fluctuations playing a substantial role in influencing oral health at various life stages, including puberty, menses, pregnancy, and menopause [34].

Menopause, a natural physiological process typically occurring around the fifth decade of a woman‘s life, marks the end of the fertile phase. During menopause, women undergo biological and endocrine changes, particularly in sex steroid hormone production, which can impact overall health [35].

The presence of estrogen receptors in the oral mucosa makes the oral cavity susceptible to direct effects from variations in hormone levels. Peri- and postmenopausal women commonly experience oral symptoms such as xerostomia, a sensation of painful mouth with numerous potential causes, and burning mouth syndrome. Understanding and addressing these oral health issues specific to women are crucial for providing comprehensive and tailored healthcare [36].

Hypovitaminosis of vitamins A, D, and C is the cause of tooth decay. Vitamin A plays a special role during the development of the dental organ and the periodontium. The lack of vitamin D manifests itself with more caries, as the calcification phase of the tooth is disturbed. Vitamin C played a special role during the development of connective tissue and collagen in the first phase of dental organ formation [13].

Calcium serves as a crucial component of the body's skeleton, and its adequate supply in the diet is essential, particularly in the context of reduced endogenous synthesis. This becomes especially important in cases of endocrine problems to support the maintenance of healthy bones and teeth [37, 38]. The body's regulation of calcium metabolism is orchestrated by vitamin D, which exerts its influence on the gastrointestinal tract, kidneys, and skeleton.

Vitamin D, a lipophilic steroid hormone, plays a significant role in oral health by acting as an anti-inflammatory agent, stimulating the production of anti-microbial peptides [39, 40]. The term “vitamin D” refers to a group of fat-soluble biomolecules synthesized in the skin through exposure to ultraviolet irradiation from the sun. Apart from its role in oral health, vitamin D is also closely associated with bone metabolism and skeletal integrity [41].

### 2.6 Food

Dental caries is a dynamic process characterized by the interaction of susceptible tooth surfaces; cariogenic bacteria, primarily *Streptococcus mutans*; and a fermentable carbohydrate source. Among dietary sugars, sucrose is the most common and is considered the most cariogenic carbohydrate. The risk of developing dental caries is heightened with frequent consumption of carbohydrates, especially in the form of simple sugars [42].

Dental caries is a multifactorial disease heavily influenced by behavioral factors, with oral hygiene, fluoride use, and dietary habits playing crucial roles [43]. Excessive consumption of fermentable carbohydrates has been identified as a primary driver, impacting the integrity of teeth as well as the pH of plaque and biofilm [44]. Beyond the quantity of carbohydrates, the frequency of carbohydrate intake is also considered a significant factor in the risk of developing dental caries [45]. Recent research has revealed positive associations between the frequency of sugar consumption and the incidence of caries, observed in both adults and children [46, 47].

Dental caries occurs when the demineralization of the enamel surpasses its demineralization capacity [42]. Bacteria present in dental plaque metabolize fermentable carbohydrates, especially sucrose, from the diet. This metabolic activity produces organic acids, leading to a decrease in pH. It is hypothesized that when the pH falls below 5.5, demineralization of the enamel occurs—a threshold known as the critical pH. This demineralization process occurs each time fermentable carbohydrates are consumed.

## 3. Local factors

### 3.1 Dental morphology

The concept of dental morphology involves the study of teeth in terms of their size, shape, and arrangement within the oral cavity. Klein and Palmer initially described the connection between dental caries and different morphological types of teeth [48]. Some characteristics of dental morphology predispose teeth to dental decay. Presently, it is recognized that most dental caries are confined to specific sites. Here are some crucial reasons for this:

#### *3.1.1 Tooth shape and size*

Molars and premolars are more susceptible to decay than other teeth due to their complex surfaces and grooves (fissures). These grooves can be deep and narrow, making it challenging for toothbrush bristles to clean effectively, leading to an accumulation of plaque and food particles, thus increasing decay risk. Mandibular molars are significantly more prone to caries than other teeth. It appears that irregularities on the occlusal surface facilitate the development of biofilm, eventually leading to carious lesions [49].

Teeth that are smaller than average may have larger gaps between them, trapping food and debris more easily, thus leading to plaque formation and an increased risk of dental caries, particularly when oral hygiene is poor. Teeth that are larger or shaped in a way that causes uneven distribution of biting forces can suffer from excessive wear. This can lead to the breakdown of enamel over time, making the teeth more susceptible to decay. Some individuals are born with congenitally misshaped teeth, or they may develop teeth of altered size due to factors like grinding (bruxism). These conditions affect the effectiveness of cleaning teeth and protecting them from decay.

#### *3.1.2 Spacing and alignment*

When teeth are crowded or misaligned, they form tight spaces that are challenging to clean properly. This difficulty can lead to plaque buildup, increasing the likelihood of cavities developing between the teeth (known as interproximal decay).

When teeth aren't properly aligned, they can wear unevenly. This misalignment can create specific niches and crannies where plaque—a sticky mix of food particles, bacteria, and saliva—tends to accumulate. If not removed in time, plaque hardens into tartar, which is much tougher to get rid of.

Misaligned teeth can also cause gum problems. Gums may not fit securely around misaligned teeth, creating pockets where bacteria can grow. This can lead to gingivitis (gum inflammation) and, if left untreated, more severe periodontal disease, which is a risk factor for tooth decay. Improper alignment can lead to abnormal wear of tooth enamel. This wear can weaken teeth and make them more susceptible to decay [50].

The gaps between teeth can trap tiny food particles, creating an ideal environment for bacteria that produce acids. These acids can erode tooth enamel, leading to cavities. For those undergoing orthodontic treatment, braces, or other appliances can make it harder to clean teeth effectively, increasing the risk of decay if proper oral hygiene is not maintained. Sometimes it is very difficult for clinicians to visualize proximal lesions during clinical exam. It is estimated that at least 40% of proximal carious lesions are missed during dental examinations [51].

Overall, while misalignment or spacing issues do not directly cause tooth decay, they create conditions that can increase the risk of decay if proper dental hygiene is not practiced.

#### *3.1.3 Enamel structure and thickness*

Variations in the thickness and quality of enamel can influence decay risk. Thinner and weaker enamel provides less protection against bacteria and acids, increasing the likelihood of tooth decay. Enamel is made up of tightly bunched, oblong crystals called crystallites, which are significantly smaller than the width of a human hair. These crystallites have a core-shell structure, where the core is more soluble than the shell. This difference in solubility can contribute to the enamel's vulnerability to decay. The core of the crystallites contains higher concentrations of impurity atoms such as magnesium, sodium, carbonate, and fluoride. These impurities, while contributing to enamel's strength, also make it more soluble, which can be a factor in tooth decay. This core-shell structure is vital for understanding the enamel's resistance and susceptibility to decay at a microscopic level [52].

Enamel thickness varies across different teeth and even within a single tooth, often being thickest at the cusp and thinnest at the borders. The thickness of enamel can be an important factor in its ability to resist decay. Thicker enamel might provide more resistance against the acidic environment in the mouth that leads to decay, whereas thinner enamel might be more susceptible to decay [52].

The atomic structure of enamel, particularly the core surrounded by shell crystallites, highlights specific areas within the teeth more prone to decay. Understanding these structures on an atomic level can lead to improved strategies for strengthening teeth against decay and repairing erosion damage. Furthermore, the distribution of minor components within the enamel crystallites, particularly the impurities at the core, offers insights into potential preventive measures against dental caries.

These discoveries open the door to new dental treatments and interventions. For example, they might lead to the development of materials or techniques that strengthen the enamel's crystalline structure or protect its more vulnerable parts. The research into the atomic structure and composition of tooth enamel provides a much deeper understanding of its vulnerabilities and strengths, which is crucial for developing more effective ways to combat tooth decay [52].

### 3.2 Oral hygiene

Oral hygiene, or rather the absence of it, can greatly contribute to tooth decay. There are a number of ways poor oral hygiene can lead to this common dental issue – tooth decay.

Dental plaque is a clear, sticky film that forms on your teeth when they are not properly cleaned of sugars and starches. Bacteria feed on these substances, creating plaque. If not regularly brushed and flossed away, plaque can build up, particularly in hard-to-reach spots [53]. In addition, if not removed, plaque can harden into tartar, which is difficult to clean and acts as a shield for bacteria. The bacteria in plaque produce acids that attack tooth enamel, leading to decay and gum disease [54]. The acids produced by bacteria in plaque lead to the demineralization of the tooth's enamel, creating tiny openings or holes—the first stage of cavities. Once the enamel is eroded, these acids can reach the dentin layer, which is softer and less resistant to acid [52].

Fluoride helps strengthen tooth enamel and can even reverse early signs of tooth decay. Not using fluoride-containing toothpaste or not getting enough fluoride from other sources leads to inadequate flouoride exposure, which can make teeth more susceptible to decay [55]. Also, poor oral hygiene can lead to gum disease (gingivitis), which can progress to a more serious form called periodontitis. This condition can expose the roots of your teeth to plaque and increase your risk of tooth decay [56].

Without regular brushing and flossing, food particles can remain in a mouth, providing a food source for bacteria. The longer these particles stay in a mouth, the more time bacteria have to produce acids that can cause decay [57]. Saliva helps wash away food particles and neutralize acids produced by bacteria. Therefore, poor oral hygiene can contribute to dry mouth conditions, which can exacerbate the risk of tooth decay.

### 3.3 Saliva

Saliva is protective to the oral hard and soft tissues since it supports the clearance of food debris and sugar, as well as contributes to the aggregation and elimination of microorganisms, thereby demonstrating a buffering capacity to neutralize acid components and promoting the remineralization of tooth enamel among other antimicrobial properties [58]. For example, many associations have been found between dental caries and salivary composition [58]. Such salivary properties may be used as biomarkers for the risk of future disease and could potentially inform interventions targeted at that risk [58, 59].

Dental caries is a highly prevalent microbial chronic dental disease that affects a greater percentage of the world's populations [60]. Dental caries is a sugar-driven biofilm-mediated oral disease characterized by the phasic demineralization and remineralization of the hard tissues of the tooth, besides being multifactoria [61].

The saliva encasing the soft and hard tissues of the craniofacial region contains some organic and inorganic components, which play a significant role in caries in the host, hence their critical role as biomarkers in the diagnosis of caries [62]. In simpler terms, dental caries occurs due to the imbalance of cariogenic microorganisms within the oral biofilm, which triggers the fermentation of available dietary carbohydrates into fermentative acids [63]. This process causes a loss of minerals in the dental hard tissues, eventually destroying tooth structure [63]. The way diet, host susceptibility, and microorganisms interact is a significant determinant of how dental caries will develop in an individual [64]. Considering that the teeth are continuously bathed in saliva, the salivary components undoubtedly play a fundamental role both in the initiation and progression of dental caries and are considered a major biomarker for the diagnosis and detection of caries.

The proteins in saliva are essential not only to maintain the integrity of the tooth but also to protect against dental caries due to various mechanisms [60]; for instance, they reduce or inhibit demineralization at the surfaces of the teeth that are exposed to this process. They are needed in the creation of a film called the acquired enamel pellicle, which provides continuous protection of the teeth from attrition and softening, as well as attracting calcium ions for the reorganization of the enamel. Nonetheless, the defense of the oral cavity also attributes to salivary proteins, including lactoferrin, proline-rich proteins, carbonic anhydrase, immunoglobulins, and mucins, which are the most common, representing about 20 to 30% of the salivary proteins [65].

## 4. Iatrogenic factors

Iatrogenic factors that cause tooth decay refer to dental decay that occurs as a result of medical or dental treatment. These factors are often unintentional and can arise from various dental procedures or treatments. Some common iatrogenic factors that can contribute to tooth decay are further explored and presented.

### 4.1 Restorative dental work

Restorative dental work, while crucial for repairing and maintaining dental health, can sometimes contribute to tooth decay if not executed or maintained properly. Sometimes, dental restorations like fillings or crowns may not fit perfectly, creating small gaps where food particles and bacteria can accumulate, leading to decay. Over time, these restorations can also wear down or break, allowing decay to develop underneath them. Restorations with margins (edges) that extend below the gum line can be challenging to clean and may irritate the surrounding gum tissue. This can lead to periodontal problems and potentially increase the risk of decay, especially at the root surfaces of teeth [66].

Dental restoration materials can degrade or wear down over time. This breakdown can lead to gaps or rough surfaces where bacteria can accumulate, increasing the risk of decay. If oral hygiene is not maintained after restorative procedures, the risk of tooth decay can increase, particularly around the restoration sites.

### 4.2 Orthodontic appliances

Braces and other orthodontic appliances can make it difficult to maintain good oral hygiene, as food particles and plaque may accumulate around brackets and wires.

Plaque is a sticky film of bacteria and food particles, and it is the primary cause of tooth decay. The complex structure of orthodontic appliances makes it more challenging to clean all areas of the teeth and gums effectively. Braces can make it harder to brush and floss effectively. This difficulty in maintaining oral hygiene can lead to a build-up of plaque and tartar, increasing the risk of tooth decay [67].

Orthodontic appliances can trap food particles, providing a constant source of nutrients for bacteria in the mouth. These bacteria produce acids that can erode tooth enamel and lead to cavities. The prolonged presence of plaque on tooth surfaces can lead to demineralization of the enamel, which is the first step in the formation of cavities. This is often seen as white spots on the teeth after braces are removed. Some orthodontic treatments or appliances might affect saliva flow in the mouth. Saliva plays a crucial role in neutralizing acids and washing away food particles, so a reduction can increase the risk of decay.

To mitigate these risks, it's important for individuals with orthodontic appliances to maintain diligent oral hygiene. This includes brushing after every meal, using a fluoride toothpaste, flossing daily (using tools like floss threaders or water flossers), and regular visits to the dentist for cleanings and check-ups. Additionally, minimizing the intake of sugary foods and drinks can reduce the risk of decay [67].

### 4.3 Fluoride overuse

Excessive fluoride, particularly during early childhood when teeth are developing, can lead to a condition called dental fluorosis. This condition is characterized by changes in the appearance of the tooth enamel, ranging from mild (white streaks) to severe (brown stains, pitting). Dental fluorosis occurs when children consume too much fluoride over a prolonged period. It's essential to use fluoride cautiously, especially with young children. They should be taught to spit out toothpaste and not swallow it. The use of fluoride mouth rinses is not recommended for children under 6 years old. In general, fluorosis is preventable by moderating fluoride intake and ensuring proper use of fluoride-containing dental products [68].

### 4.4 Medications affecting saliva production

Certain medications prescribed for unrelated medical conditions can reduce saliva flow, leading to dry mouth or xerostomia [69–71]. Medications that can reduce saliva production are:

- Antihistamines: often used for allergies, they can decrease saliva flow.
- Antidepressants: some types of antidepressants can have a drying effect on the mouth.
- Antihypertensives: used to treat high blood pressure, these can also reduce saliva production.
- Diuretics: prescribed for conditions like hypertension and some kidney disorders, diuretics can decrease saliva by increasing urine production.
- Chemotherapy drugs: used in cancer treatment, some of them can affect saliva glands.

Saliva is crucial for neutralizing acids in the mouth and washing away food particles, so a reduction in saliva can increase the risk of decay [69–71].

### 4.5 Inadequate dental sealants or fluoride treatments

If dental sealants, which are meant to protect the grooves and pits in the chewing surfaces of teeth, are not applied properly or completely, they can leave parts of the tooth surface exposed to plaque and decay. Fluoride treatments help strengthen enamel and make it more resistant to acid attacks from bacteria. Inadequate application, poor quality, or insufficient frequency of fluoride treatments can reduce their effectiveness, leaving teeth more vulnerable to decay. It's important to ensure that sealants and fluoride treatments are applied correctly and monitored regularly for maintenance, to maximize their protective benefits against tooth decay [72].

### 4.6 Poor infection control

Inadequate infection control during dental procedures can lead to bacterial contamination and subsequent tooth decay. Infection control is crucial in dental clinics to prevent the spread of infectious diseases among patients and healthcare workers. This includes proper sterilization of dental instruments, use of personal protective equipment, and adherence to hygiene protocols. While lapses in these practices do not cause cavities, they can increase the risk of transmitting bacterial, viral, or fungal infections, which could complicate overall oral health and treatment outcomes [73].

## 5. Conclusions

The extensive exploration of factors influencing dental caries reveals a multifaceted and intricate nature of this dental issue. The discussion spanned various dimensions, including general factors like heredity, gender, age, immunological factors, hormones, vitamins, and diet, all contributing uniquely to the susceptibility and manifestation of dental caries.

General factors like genetics, hormonal changes, and dietary habits underscore the complexity of caries, highlighting the interplay of internal and external influences. Hereditary factors point to a genetic predisposition, while gender-related aspects, such as hormonal fluctuations in women, add another layer to the risk of caries. Age-related changes in dental structures and the immune system further accentuate the variability of caries occurrence among different age groups.

Local factors, particularly dental morphology, emphasize the significance of physical attributes of teeth in caries development. Variations in tooth shape, size, and enamel structure can increase the risk of decay, underscoring the importance of individualized dental care. Misalignments and spacing issues, although not direct causes of decay, create conditions conducive to bacterial growth and acid production, thereby increasing decay risk.

Oral hygiene practices play a pivotal role in preventing or accelerating caries development. Poor oral hygiene leads to plaque and tartar buildup, gum diseases, and enamel demineralization, which are primary contributors to tooth decay. Saliva, a key element in oral health, aids in neutralizing acids and preventing caries, with its composition and flow rate being critical in maintaining oral health.

Iatrogenic factors remind us that medical and dental interventions, though necessary, can sometimes inadvertently contribute to caries. Dental restorations, orthodontic appliances, and fluoride treatments, if not properly managed, can lead to conditions favorable for caries development.

This comprehensive analysis of caries etiology suggests that effective prevention and management strategies should be holistic, considering the interplay of genetic, environmental, behavioral, and clinical factors. It highlights the need for personalized dental care approaches, tailored to individual risk factors and specific dental characteristics. Moreover, it underscores the importance of continuous research and innovation in dental sciences to develop more effective preventive and therapeutic strategies against dental caries.

In summary, the fight against dental caries requires a multifaceted approach, integrating knowledge from various disciplines and considering the unique circumstances of each individual. This holistic understanding is crucial in developing more effective, personalized strategies for the prevention and treatment of this prevalent dental issue.

## Author details

Merita Barani-Sveçla* and Shqipe Buleshkaj
UBT College, Prishtina, Kosova

*Address all correspondence to: merita.barani@ubt-uni.net

## References

[1] Selwitz RH, Ismail AI, Pitts NB. Dental caries. The Lancet. 2007;**369**(9555):51-59

[2] Rugg-Gunn AJ, Do L. Effect of dietary sugars on dental caries incidence. British Dental Journal. 2012;**213**(11):505-510

[3] Marsh PD. Dental plaque as a biofilm and a microbial community – Implications for health and disease. BMC Oral Health. 2006;**6**(S1):S14

[4] Fejerskov O, Kidd E, editors. Dental Caries: The Disease and its Clinical Management. 3rd ed. Oxford: Wiley-Blackwell; 2015

[5] König KG. Diet and oral health. International Dental Journal. 2002;**52**(3):162-167

[6] Moynihan P. The role of diet and nutrition in the etiology and prevention of oral diseases. Bulletin of the World Health Organization. 2005;**83**(9):694-699

[7] Berkowitz RJ. Mutans streptococci: Acquisition and transmission. Pediatric Dentistry. 2003;**25**(2):106-109

[8] Zero DT. Dentifrices, mouthwashes, and remineralization/caries arrestment strategies. BMC Oral Health. 2006;**6**(S1):S9

[9] Bagramian RA, Garcia-Godoy F, Volpe AR. The global increase in dental caries. A pending public health crisis. American Journal of Dentistry. 2009;**22**(1):3-8

[10] American Dental Association. Caries Risk Assessment and Management. Chicago, IL: ADA; 2020

[11] Green S, Higgins JPT, Alderson P, Clarke M, Mulrow CD, Oxman AD. Cochrane Handbook for Systematic Review of Interventions. Chichester, West Sussex, England: John Wiley & Sons Ltd; 2011

[12] Borenstein M, Hedges LV, Higgins JPT, Rothstein HR. Introduction to Meta-Analysis. Chichester, West Sussex, United Kingdom: John Wiley & Sons Ltd; 2009

[13] Hoxha V. Etiopatogjeneza e kariesit; Semundjet e dhembit. Prishtina, Kosovo; 2019. pp. 54-59

[14] Opal S, Garg S, Jain J, Walia I. Genetics factors affecting dental caries risk. Australian Dental Journal. 2015;**60**(1):2-11. DOI: 10.1111/adj.12262

[15] Mosaddad SA, Tahmasebi E, Yazdanian A, Rezvani MB, Seifalian A, Yazdanian M, et al. Oral microbial biofilms: Un update. European Journal of Clinical Microbiology & Infectious Diseases. 2019;**38**(11):2005-2019. DOI: 10.1007/s10096-019-03641-9. Epub 2019

[16] Li Z, Hu X, Zhou J, Xie X, Zhang J. Genetic polymorphisms in the carbonic anhydrase VI gene and dental caries susceptibility. Genetics and Molecular Research. 2015;**14**(2):5986-5993. DOI: 10.4238/2015.June.1.16

[17] Izakovicova Holla L, Borilova Linhartova P, Kastovsky J, Bartosova M, Musilova K, Kukla L, et al. Vitamin D receptor Taq i gene polymorphism and dental caries in Czech children. Caries Research. 2017;**51**(1):7-11. DOI: 10.1159/000452635

[18] Chai CK, Hunt HR, Hoppert CA, Rosen S. Hereditary basis of caries resistance in rats. Journal of Dental

Research. 1968;**47**(1):127-138. DOI: 10.1177/00220345680470010601

[19] Werneck RI, Mira MT, Trevilatto PC. A critical review: An overview of genetic influence on dental caries. Oral Diseases. 2010;**16**(7):613-623. DOI: 10.1111/j.1601-0825.2010.01675.x

[20] Telatar G, Ermiş B. Çürük riski ve genetik. Journal of Dental Faculty of Atatürk University. 2019;**29**(2):350-356. DOI: 10.17567/ataunidfd.289346

[21] Lukacs JR. Sex differences in dental caries experience: Clinical evidence, complex etiology. Clinical Oral Investigations. 2011;**15**:649-656

[22] Lukacs JR, Largaespada LL. Explaining sex differences in dental caries prevalence: Saliva, hormones, and 'life history' etiologies. American Journal of Human Biology. 2006;**18**(4):540-555

[23] Martinez-Mier EA, Zandona AF. The impact of gender on caries prevalence and risk assessment. Dental Clinics of North America. 2013;**57**(2):301-315

[24] Lipsky MS, Su S, Crespo CJ, Hung M. Men and oral health: A review of sex and gender differences. American Journal of Men's Health. May-Jun 2021;**15**(3):15579883211016361

[25] Mamai-Homata E, Koletsi-Kounari H, Margaritis V. Gender differences in oral health status and behavior of Greek dental students: A meta-analysis of 1981, 2000, and 2010 data. Journal of International Society of Preventive & Community Dentistry. 2016;**6**(1):60-68

[26] Kateeb E. Gender-specific oral health attitudes and behaviour among dental students in Palestine. Eastern Mediterranean Health Journal. 2010;**16**(3):329-333

[27] McGrath C, Bedi R. Gender variations in the social impact of oral health. Journal of the Irish Dental Association. 2000;**46**(3):87-91

[28] Bäck K, Hakeberg M, Wide U, Hange D, Dahlström L. Orofacial pain and its relationship with oral health-related quality of life and psychological distress in middle-aged women. Acta Odontologica Scandinavica. 2020;**78**(1):74-80

[29] Furuta M, Ekuni D, Irie K, et al. Sex differences in gingivitis relate to interaction of oral health behaviors in young people. Journal of Periodontology. 2011;**82**(4):558-565

[30] Lamster IB, Asadourian L, Del Carmen T, Friedman PK. The aging mouth: Differentiating normal aging from disease. Periodontology 2000. 2016;**72**(1):96-107. DOI: 10.1111/prd.12131

[31] Setia S, Gambhir RS, Kapoor V. Immunology in prevention of dental caries. Universal research. Journal of Dentistry. 2012;**2**(2):58-63

[32] Stephens MB, Wiedemer JP, Kushner GM. Dental problem in primary care. American Family Physician. 2018;**98**(11):654-660

[33] Sampaio-Maia B, Caldas IM, Pereira ML, Pérez-Mongiovi D, Araujo R. The oral microbiome in health and its implication in ral and systemic diseases. Advances in Applied Microbiology. 2016;**97**:171-210. DOI: 10.1016/bs.aambs.2016.08.002. Epub 2016 Sep 21

[34] August M. Oral health implications of menopause. Menopause. 2005;**12**:123-124

[35] Frutos R, Rodríguez S, Miralles-Jorda L, Machuca G. Oral

manifestations and dental treatment in menopause. Medicina Oral. 2002;**7**:26-35

[36] Meurman JH, Tarkkila L, Tiitinen A. The menopause and oral health. Maturitas. 2009;**63**:56-62

[37] Bhale DV, Ansari HA. Study of serum calcium levels in postmenopausal women of Aurangabad district. International Journal of Recent Trends in Science and Technology. 2014;**9**(3):332-333

[38] Patwa CK, Jindani N, Afroz S. Study of serum calcium levels in premenopausal women and postmenopausal women. Med Pulse International Journal of Physiology. 2017;**4**(2):14-16

[39] Pérez-López FR, Brincat M, Erel CT, et al. EMAS position statement: Vitamin D and postmenopausal health. Maturitas. 2012;**71**:83-88

[40] Uwitonze AM, Murererehe J, Ineza MC, et al. Effects of vitamin D status on oral health. The Journal of Steroid Biochemistry and Molecular Biology. 2018;**175**:190-194

[41] Hamdi AQ, Sarhat ER, Ali NH, Sarhat TR. Evaluation of Lipocalin-2 and visfatin, and vitamin (D, C, and E) in serum of diabetic patients with chronic periodontitis. Indian Journal of Forensic Medicine & Toxicology. 2021;**15**(2):1668-1674

[42] Tungare S, Paranjpe AG. Diet and nutrition to prevent dental problems. In: StatPearls. Treasure Island (FL): StatPearls Publishing; 2023 [Accessed: Jul 10, 2023]

[43] WHO. Guideline: Sugars Intake for Adults and Children. Geneva: WHO; 2015

[44] Twetman S. Prevention of dental caries as a non-communicable disease. European Journal of Oral Sciences. 2018;**126**(Suppl. 1):19-25

[45] van Loveren C. Sugar restriction for caries prevention: Amount and frequency. Which is more important? Caries Research. 2019;**53**(2):168-175

[46] Bernabé E, Vehkalahti MM, Sheiham A, Lundqvist A, Suominen AL. The shape of the dose-response relationship between sugars and caries in adults. Journal of Dental Research. 2016;**95**(2):167-172

[47] Dusseldorp E, Kamphuis M, Schuller A. Impact of lifestyle factors on caries experience in three different age groups: 9, 15, and 21-year-olds. Community Dentistry and Oral Epidemiology. 2015;**43**(1):9-16

[48] Klein H, Palmer CE. Studies on dental caries. XI. Comparison of the caries susceptibility of the various morphological types of permanent teeth. Journal of Dental Research. 1941;**20**:203-216

[49] Carvalho JC, Ekstrand KR, Thylstrup A. Dental plaque and caries on occlusal surfaces of first permanent molars in relation to stage of eruption. Journal of Dental Research. 1989;**68**(5):773-779. DOI: 10.1177/00220345890680050401

[50] Lynch RJ. The primary and mixed dentition, post-eruptive enamel maturation and dental caries: A review. International Dental Journal. 2013;**63**(Suppl. 2):3-13. DOI: 10.1111/idj.12076

[51] Ricketts D, Kidd E, Weerheijm K, de Soet H. Hidden caries: What is it? Does it exist? Does it matter? International Dental Journal. 1997;**47**(5):259-265. DOI: 10.1002/j.1875-595x.1997.tb00786.x

[52] Hicks J, Garcia-Godoy F, Flaitz C. Biological factors in dental caries enamel

structure and the caries process in the dynamic process of demineralization and remineralization (part 2). The Journal of Clinical Pediatric Dentistry. 2004;**28**(2):119-124. DOI: 10.17796/jcpd.28.2.617404w302446411

[53] Marsh PD. Microbiology of dental plaque biofilms and their role in oral health and caries. Dental Clinics of North America. 2010;**54**(3):441-454. DOI: 10.1016/j.cden.2010.03.002

[54] Huynh HT, Verneau J, Levasseur A, Drancourt M, Aboudharam G. Bacteria and archaea paleomicrobiology of the dental calculus: A review. Molecular Oral Microbiology. 2016;**31**(3):234-242. DOI: 10.1111/omi.12118

[55] Whelton HP, Spencer AJ, Do LG, Rugg-Gunn AJ. Fluoride revolution and dental caries: Evolution of policies for global use. Journal of Dental Research. 2019;**98**(8):837-846. DOI: 10.1177/0022034519843495

[56] Löe H. Oral hygiene in the prevention of caries and periodontal disease. International Dental Journal. 2000;**50**(3):129-139. DOI: 10.1111/j.1875-595x.2000.tb00553.x

[57] Hujoel PP, Hujoel MLA, Kotsakis GA. Personal oral hygiene and dental caries: A systematic review of randomised controlled trials. Gerodontology. 2018;**35**(4):282-289. DOI: 10.1111/ger.12331

[58] Gao X, Jiang S, Koh D, Hsu CY. Salivary biomarkers for dental caries. Periodontology 2000. 2016;**70**:128-141

[59] Javaid MA, Ahmed AS, Durand R, Tran SD. Saliva as a diagnostic tool for oral and systemic diseases. Journal of Oral Biology and Craniofacial Research. 2016;**6**:66-75

[60] Hicks J, Garcia-Godoy F, Flaitz C. Biological factors in dental caries: Role of saliva and dental plaque in the dynamic process of demineralization and remineralization (part 1). The Journal of Clinical Pediatric Dentistry. 2003;**28**:47-52

[61] Pitts NB, Zero DT, Marsh PD, Ekstrand K, Weintraub JA, Ramos-Gomez F, et al. Dental caries. Nature Reviews. Disease Primers. 2017;**3**:17030

[62] Ahsan H. Biomolecules and biomarkers in oral cavity: Bioassays and immunopathology. Journal of Immunoassay and Immunochemistry. 2019;**40**:52-69

[63] Chen X, Daliri EB-M, Kim N, Kim J-R, Yoo D, Oh D-H. Microbial etiology and prevention of dental caries: Exploiting natural products to inhibit cariogenic biofilms. Pathogens. 2020;**9**:569

[64] Subiksha PS, Sandhya R. Salivary biomarkers in diagnosis of dental caries—A review article. International Journal of Dentistry and Oral Science. 2021;**8**:3729-3733

[65] Pedersen L, Belstrøm D. The role of natural salivary defences in maintaining a healthy oral microbiota. Journal of Dentistry. 2019;**80**:S3-S12

[66] Reddy KV, Nirupama C, Reddy PK, Koppolu P, Alotaibi DH. Effect of iatrogenic factors on periodontal health: An epidemiological study. The Saudi Dental Journal. 2020;**32**(2):80-85. DOI: 10.1016/j.sdentj.2019.07.001

[67] Lazar L, Vlasa A, Beresescu L, Bud A, Lazar AP, Matei L, et al. White spot lesions (WSLs)-post-orthodontic occurrence, management and treatment alternatives: A narrative review. Journal

of Clinical Medicine. 2023;**12**(5):1908. DOI: 10.3390/jcm12051908

[68] Zotti F, Albertini L, Tomizioli N, Capocasale G, Albanese M. Resin infiltration in dental fluorosis treatment-1-year follow-up. Medicina (Kaunas, Lithuania). 2020;**57**(1):22. DOI: 10.3390/medicina57010022

[69] Kawamoto M, Yamada SI, Gibo T, Kajihara R, Nagashio S, Tanaka H, et al. Relationship between dry mouth and hypertension. Clinical Oral Investigations. 2021;**25**(9):5217-5225. DOI: 10.1007/s00784-021-03829-4

[70] Tanasiewicz M, Hildebrandt T, Obersztyn I. Xerostomia of various etiologies: A review of the literature. Advances in Clinical and Experimental Medicine: Official Organ Wroclaw Medical University. 2016;**25**(1):199-206. DOI: 10.17219/acem/29375

[71] Tan ECK, Lexomboon D, Sandborgh-Englund G, Haasum Y, Johnell K. Medications that cause dry mouth as an adverse effect in older people: A systematic review and metaanalysis. Journal of the American Geriatrics Society. 2018;**66**(1):76-84. DOI: 10.1111/jgs.15151

[72] Deery C, Fyffe HE, Nugent Z, Nuttall NM, Pitts NB. Integrity, maintenance and caries susceptibility of sealed surfaces in adolescents receiving regular care from general dental practitioners in Scotland. International Journal of Paediatric Dentistry. 1997;**7**(2):75-80. DOI: 10.1111/j.1365-263x.1997.tb00282.x

[73] Coll PP, Lindsay A, Meng J, Gopalakrishna A, Raghavendra S, Bysani P, et al. The prevention of infections in older adults: Oral health. Journal of the American Geriatrics Society. 2020;**68**(2):411-416. DOI: 10.1111/jgs.16154

Chapter 2

# Enamel and Its Interaction with the Oral Environment

*Sittichai Koontongkaew, Kusumawadee Utispan, Darren Dhananthat Chawhuaveang, Ollie Yiru Yu and Rattapong Worawongvasu*

## Abstract

Enamel, comprised of hydroxyapatite (HAP) units forming crystallites and rods, constitutes the structure of teeth. HAP is represented by the stoichiometric formula $Ca_{10}(PO_4)_6(OH)_2$. However, biological HAP, found in enamel, deviates from this stoichiometry due to deficiencies in $Ca^{2+}$, $PO_4^{3-}$, and $OH^-$, and contamination with $CO_3^{2-}$ and $HPO_4^{2-}$, and trace elements within their lattice. Its integrity is influenced by saliva, oral bacteria, fluoride from oral care products, and dietary acids. Salivary glycoproteins form an acquired salivary pellicle on enamel, while oral microorganisms create dental biofilm, which can become cariogenic with increased sucrose levels. The cariogenic biofilm generates acids, which reduces hydroxyl and phosphate groups surrounding enamel, thereby lowering the ion activity product (Ip) of the dental biofilm fluid and saliva and resulting in enamel demineralization. Initial caries appear as subsurface lesions with crystallite dissolution, mitigated by topical fluoride promoting the formation of calcium fluoride-like reservoirs on tooth surfaces and within dental biofilm. Enamel becomes susceptible to irreversible wear with frequent and prolonged dietary acid exposure. Dental erosion, chemically induced below pH 4.5, dissolves fluorapatite and hydroxyapatite predominantly on the surface layer, without subsurface lesions. Understanding these processes is crucial for preventive strategies against dental caries and erosion.

**Keywords:** enamel rod, hydroxyapatite, the oral environment, acquired salivary pellicle, dental biofilm, dental caries, fluoride, dental erosion

## 1. Introduction

Enamel is an incredibly remarkable mineralized tissue that not only covers the exterior surfaces of teeth but also significantly contributes to our overall appearance and plays a vital role in digestion. Its organizational complexity spans multiple dimensions, ranging from the atomic level with hydroxyapatite (HAP) units to structures at the micrometer level such as crystallites, up to the millimeter level including enamel rods, and finally encompassing the entirety of the tooth surface. In the oral cavity, enamel interacts with the surrounding aqueous environment, which consists of saliva, oral bacteria, fluoride sourced from oral care products, and dietary acids. Consequently, the conditions within the oral cavity can be quite harsh environmentally, presenting biological and chemical challenges to the integrity of enamel. As a crucial component in the initial stages of digestion, the enamel is exposed to a variety of both protective and harmful agents as part of the dentition's function.

The acquired salivary pellicle is mainly formed by the selective adsorption of salivary glycoproteins and proteins from various sources, primarily saliva. In addition to providing protection against enamel demineralization, the pellicle also serves as a foundation for the subsequent development of dental biofilm. The mouth harbors a diverse range of oral microorganisms that form biofilms on dental and mucosal surfaces. These resident oral bacteria contribute to host defenses by hindering the establishment of many exogenous microorganisms. The development of dental biofilm can be categorized into several stages, with numerous non-specific and specific interactions occurring between the pellicle and bacterial cells, ultimately determining the success of attachment and colonization.

Despite dental biofilms being natural and contributing to host well-being, on occasion, this symbiotic relationship can deteriorate, leading to oral diseases. Several hypotheses regarding the development of dental caries and periodontal diseases were proposed during the nineteenth and twentieth centuries. However, the Ecological Plaque Hypothesis (EPH) has gained widespread acceptance. According to this hypothesis, the disease results from an imbalance in the total microbiota due to ecological stress, leading to an enrichment of certain oral pathogens or disease-related microorganisms in dental biofilm. Dental caries is a multifactorial disease greatly influenced by the host's diet, making it a fitting example for the EPH. Individuals who frequently consume significant amounts of fermentable carbohydrates are selected for acidogenic and aciduric bacteria that lead to acid production. In the cariogenic environment, both $OH^-$ and $PO_4^{3-}$ ions are reduced, consequently lowering the Ip to a value often below the solubility product constant (Ksp), resulting in enamel dissolution. Remineralization, an important natural repair process, counteracts cariogenic challenges to maintain the balance between mineral loss and gain. Therefore, the caries process entails the accumulation of numerous episodes of demineralization and remineralization, rather than a unidirectional demineralization process.

Currently, it is known that fluoride ions fit well into the structure of a HAP crystal, even better than the hydroxyl group, resulting in lower solubility of fluorapatite (FAP) compared to HAP. However, many studies indicate that a compound similar to calcium fluoride ($CaF_2$) is an important source of fluoride for oral fluids. This compound forms when the fluoride concentration in the solution surrounding the enamel surface exceeds 100 ppmF. Therefore, given the high fluoride concentration in oral care products, it is expected that a calcium fluoride-like reservoir forms on tooth surfaces, primarily within dental biofilm. Finally, it should be noted that fluoride ions can adsorb to the surface of sound enamel and/or partially demineralized crystallites, attracting calcium ions and enhancing remineralization.

Enamel has inherent mechanisms to counteract daily exposure to dietary acids. Consequently, repeated contact with dietary acids, particularly over prolonged durations, can result in dental erosion. Dental erosion is identified by the deterioration of dental hard tissue *via* a non-bacterial chemical process. This degradation can be initiated by either hydrogen ions or chelating agents. Typically, dental erosion happens when the pH of fluids around the tooth drops below 4.5, leading to the dissolution of both FAP and HAP in such acidic environments.

## 2. Chemical compositions and structural hierarchy of enamel

The mineral content of enamel includes HAP, calcium carbonate, calcium fluoride, and magnesium phosphate, making up around 89, 4, 2, and 1.5% of its makeup, respectively [1]. Enamel is composed of 17.7 wt % phosphorus, 36.5 wt % calcium, 3.5 wt % carbonate, 0.5 wt % sodium, 0.44 wt % magnesium, 0.3 wt % chloride, and 0.01% fluoride [2]. Three of the classic enamel proteins including amelogenin, ameloblastin, and enamelin are known to be essential to form tooth enamel. However, a small amount of protein remains in tooth enamel after mineralization is completed and teeth are erupted [3]. Enamel, the toughest biological material found in humans, is formed by specialized cells known as ameloblasts. Within its histological structure, enamel comprises enamel rods (also called prisms) and interrods, serving as the basic building blocks of tooth enamel (**Figure 1**). Enamel rods, cylindrical-like structures measuring 5–8 μm in diameter, traverse the entire width of the enamel from the dentino-enamel junction (DEJ) to the outer surface of the tooth. A thin rod sheath surrounds each rod and separates it from adjacent rods by an interrod substance [4]. The rod is shaped somewhat like a cylinder and made up of HAP crystallites or crystals (**Figure 2**).

The crystal is the true structural unit of enamel. The smallest space unit of the HAP crystals is called the hydroxyapatite unit cell [$Ca_{10}(PO_4)_6(OH)_2$], containing 10 calcium ions, 6 phosphate ions, and 2 hydroxyl ions [5]. Every enamel rod is composed of millions of HAP crystallites, measuring approximately 70 nm in width and 30 nm in thickness, and varying in length. A distinguishing characteristic of mature enamel crystallites is their significant size compared to those found in dentine, cementum, and bone [6–8]. When viewed in cross section, enamel rods display a pattern resembling fish scales or keyholes, comprising a head and a tail (**Figure 3**). The head of each rod is defined by a slender proteinaceous sheath, approximately 0.5 μm in thickness. Densely packed HAP crystals were organized into enamel rods. Crystallites in the head region align along the long axis of the rod, while those in the tail align perpendicular to the head (**Figure 4**) [7, 9, 10]. It is crucial to highlight that the "keyhole" pattern is considered within the context of the classic concept. Notably, the rod tail exhibits less distinct boundaries and seamlessly transitions into the interrod enamel [11].

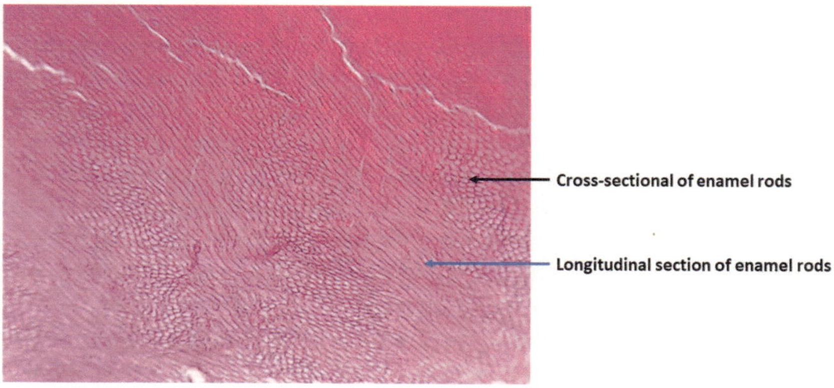


**Figure 1.**
*A light micrograph of forming enamel rods. Hematoxylin and eosin staining shows the row of numbered enamel rods forming as a wavy course. One part is cut longitudinally (blue arrow), while another part is cut cross-sectionally (black arrow) (the photograph was kindly provided by the Department of Oral Biology, Faculty of Dentistry, Thammasat University, Thailand).*

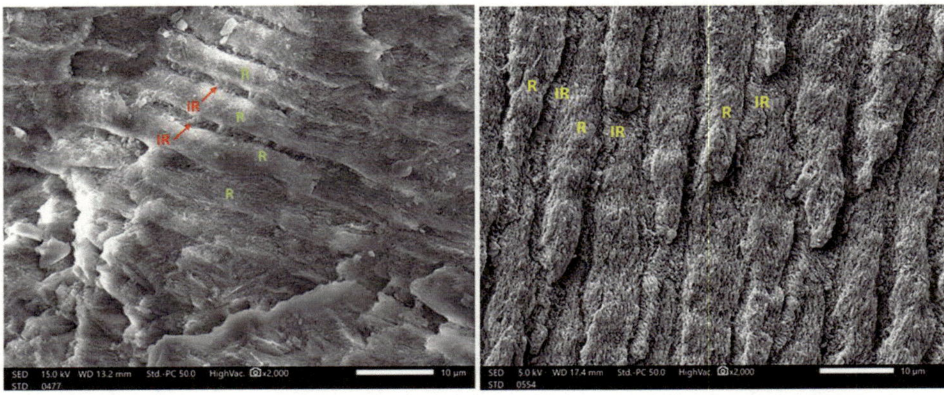


(A) (B)

**Figure 2.**
*Longitudinal-sectioned scanning electron microscopy (SEM) image of human enamel rods. (A) Enamel is constructed via cylindrical enamel rods (R) and interrod enamel (IR). Each enamel rod is composed of numerous HAP crystallites (original magnification x 2000). (B) Densely packed HAP crystallites were organized into enamel rods (R) and interrods (IR). Notably, the interrod surrounds each rod, and its crystallites are oriented in a direction different from those making up the enamel rod (original magnification x 2000) (Courtesy: Dr. Apiwat Ridhabhaya, International College of Dentistry, Walailak University, Bangkok, Thailand).*

Fundamentally, in longitudinal section, enamel prisms are cylindrical, making the term "rods" more accurate [9, 12]. Despite the enamel rod not strictly conforming to a prismatic outline, the term "enamel prism" has gained acceptance through widespread usage [6].

The crystals within the enamel rod exhibit no variation in size, shape, and composition when compared to those in the interrod region. When crystallites are generated from the distal end of the Tomes' process, they align parallel to the rod axis. Nonetheless, the alignment of crystallites varies when they originate from the proximal part of the Tomes' process (**Figure 5**) [13]. Given that the distal and proximal ends of the Tomes' process are angled at approximately 30 degrees, the crystallites in both the rod and interrod enamel also display this angular orientation [8, 9, 14]. Each individual crystallite is stacked atop another and held together by a thin layer, approximately 2 nm thick, of hydrated protein. These enamel crystallites, in turn, constitute a self-assembled agglomeration of HAP nanoparticles, ranging in size from 20 to 40 nm, which serve as the fundamental building blocks of enamel. The HAP nanoparticles maintain cohesion through more rigid, interfacial molecular bonds, including hydrogen bonds facilitated by surface-hydrated water molecules (**Figure 6**) [15–17].

The building block unit of enamel, dentine, cementum, and bone corresponded to an apatite structure. Generally, stoichiometric HAP, which is $Ca_{10}(PO_4)_6(OH)_2$, has been used as a model of tooth and bone minerals [18]. Ten $Ca^{2+}$ ions (20 positive charges), six $PO_4^{3-}$ ions (18 negative charges), and two $OH^-$ ions (2 negative charges) in $Ca_{10}(PO_4)_6(OH)_2$ hold together by electrostatic interactions [19, 20]. The spatial arrangement of HAP atoms is intricate, and a detailed configuration is beyond the scope of this chapter. Here, we present only the fundamental elements of the structure. Basically, isolated HAP unit cells cannot exist independently and are associated with numerous repeating units in a crystallite. **Figure 7** illustrates a three-dimensional concept of the HAP unit cell within a crystal. The a-b axes lie in the same plane, forming the floor and ceiling of a parallelogram, with each side measuring 0.942 nm

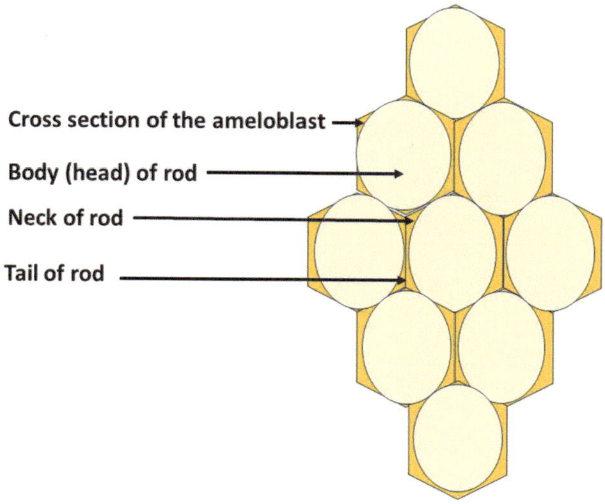


**Figure 3.**
*Schematic representation of the keyhole concept of enamel rod. The diagram shows the six-sided ameloblasts overlying keyhole-shaped enamel. Body (head), neck, and tail of the enamel rod are also shown in the diagram.*

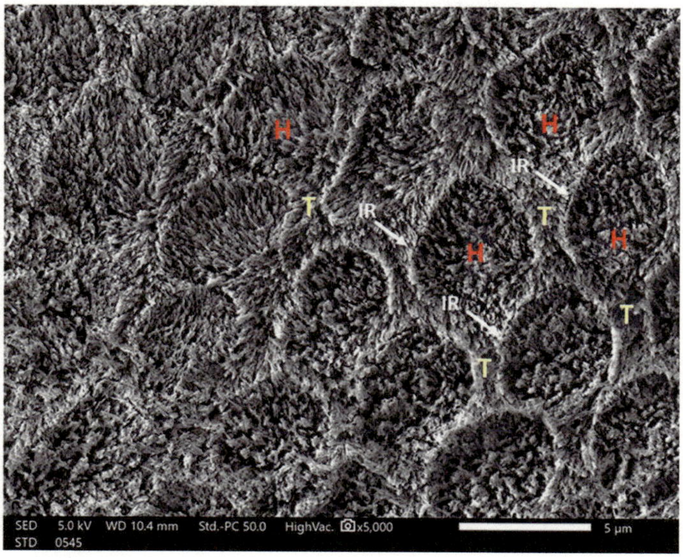


**Figure 4.**
*Cross-sectioned SEM image of human enamel rods. The image was obtained by SEM (original magnification X 5000). Head (H) and tail (T) in keyhole-like patterns of enamel rods were observed in this figure. Notably, interrod enamel (IR) is located around each enamel rod, and it enhances the "keyhole" appearance of enamel rods by acting as its border (Courtesy: Dr. Apiwat Ridhabhaya, International College of Dentistry, Walailak University, Bangkok, Thailand).*

and two angles each of 60 and 120°. The height of the unit cell (0.688 nm) aligns in the c-axis, perpendicular to the a-b plane and parallel to the long axis of the crystal [5, 21].

The phosphates within each HAP unit cell are separated into two layers, with heights of 0.25c and 0.75c, as illustrated in **Figure 8**. These layers predominantly fill the space and form the essential framework of the unit cell. According to the

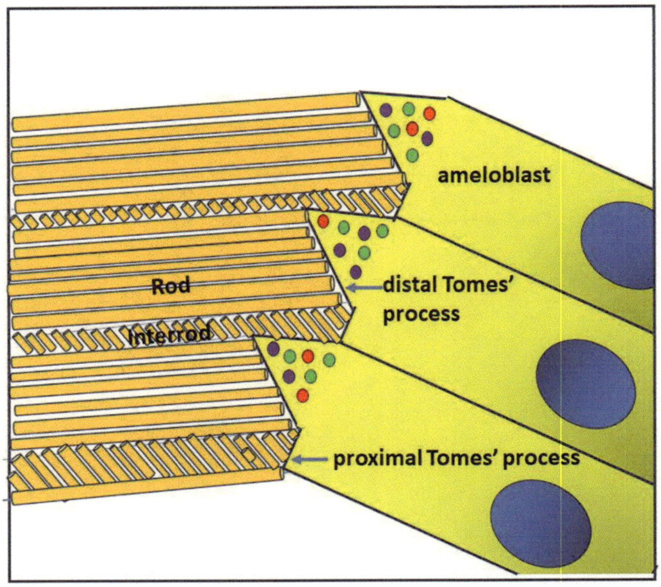


**Figure 5.**
*Schematic representation of secretory ameloblasts. The organization of secretory ameloblasts as would be revealed in a section along their long axis. Prismatic enamel rod is produced by the distal end of Tomes' process, and interprismatic enamel ("interrod") by proximal portions of the Tomes' process. Red, purple, and green dots in the Tomes' process represented secretory granules in ameloblasts.*

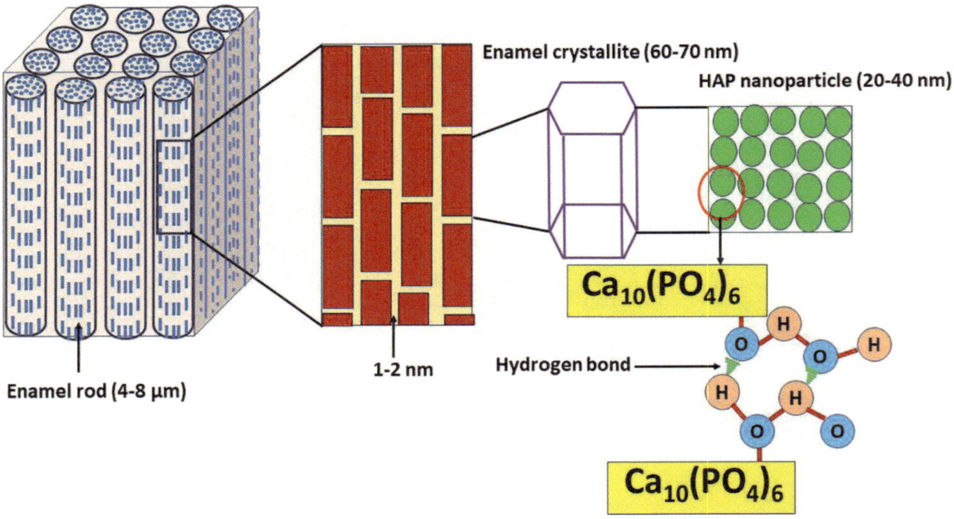


**Figure 6.**
*Schematic representation of the nanostructure of enamel crystallites. Each enamel rod (4–8 µm in size) consists of many crystallites approximately 60–70 nm wide. Individual crystallite is stacked one on top of another and "glued" together by a thin layer (approximately 1–2 nm thick) of hydrated protein. Each enamel crystallite is, in turn, a self-assembled agglomeration of HAP nanoparticles (20–40 nm), which are the basic building blocks of enamel. The HAP nanoparticles hold together with more rigid, interfacial molecular bonds including hydrogen bonds (Adapted from Ref. [15]).*

difference in calcium ion position, the general formula of HAP is Ca-$I_4$Ca-$II_6$ $(PO_4)_6(OH)_2$, where Ca-I and Ca-II are two different crystallographic positions for 10 calcium atoms. Four of them are situated in the Ca-I position, and the other

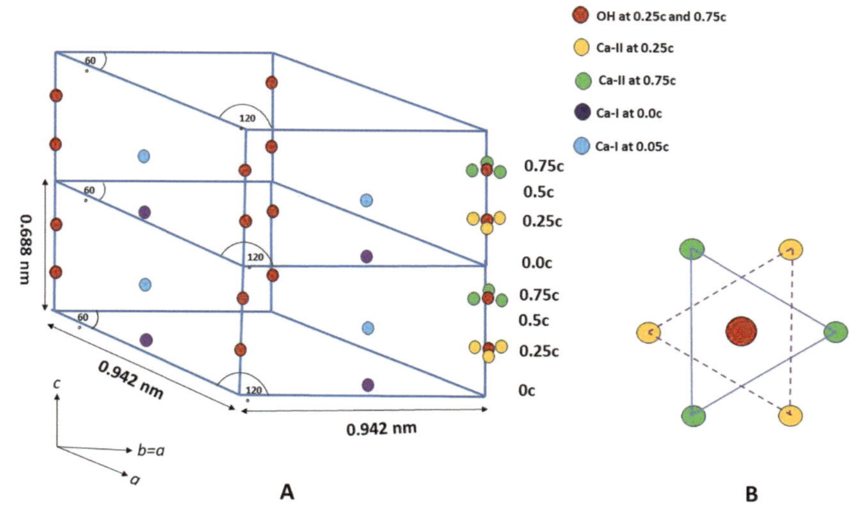


**Figure 7.**
*Schematic representation of hydroxyapatite unit cell. (A) The unit cell of HAP projected along a-axis. The a- and b-axes form a parallelogram with each side 0.942 nm. The height represents the c-axes and is 0.688 nm. Note two hydroxyl groups are located at 0.25c and 0.75c of the height of unit cells. Calcium ions (II) are also located in the screw axis at 0.25c and 0.75c in the form of equilateral triangles around the two hydroxyl groups. Calcium ions (I) are located inside the unit cell at the a-b plane (0.0c) and one-half the distance between the two a-b planes (0.5c). (B) The unit cell of HAP projected along c-axes. Diagram illustration of stacking of Ca-II ions in the form of equilateral triangles around the hydroxyl groups. The adjacent triangle does not line at the same plane but are rotated by 180 degrees with respect to each other. Notably, when viewing along the c-axis, the hydroxyl ions are exactly superimposed. Phosphate groups are omitted in the diagrams for clarity.*

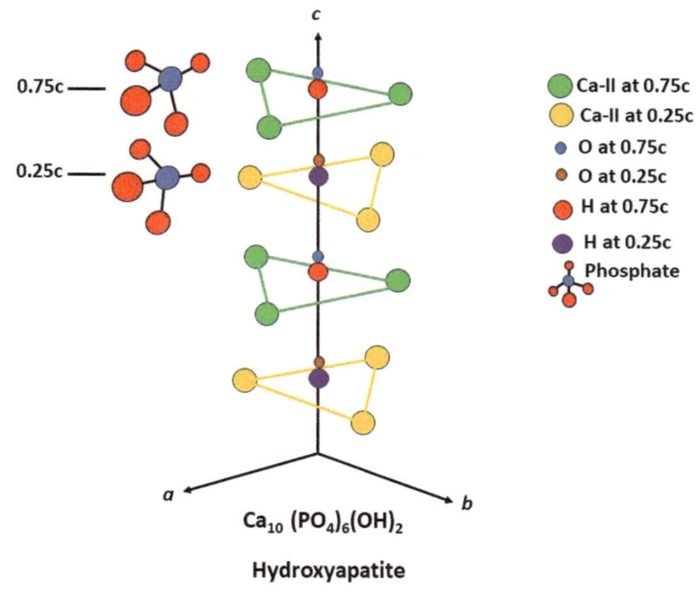


**Figure 8.**
*Schematic representation of the position of phosphate tetrahedral groups with respect to the c-axis. Hydroxyl ions located in the central c-axis at 0.25c and 0.75c are surrounded by calcium-II, phosphates, and Ca-I. Calcium-II ions surrounded the screw axis at 0.25c and 0.75c. Six Ca-II ions are situated on two oppositely directed triangles perpendicular to the c-axis and separated by 0.5c. At a slightly greater distance, one finds phosphate groups similarly arranged. Notably, hydroxyl ions, Ca-II ions, and phosphate groups are shown in this figure, whereas Ca-I ions are omitted for clarity.*

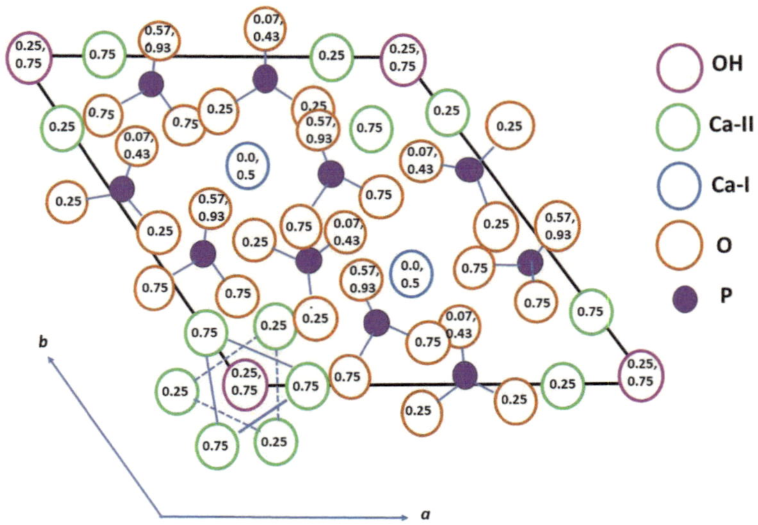


**Figure 9.**
*Hydroxyapatite lattice structure projected along the c-axis. The number written in the symbol is z parameter (direction perpendicular to the page) (Adapted from Ref. [24]).*

six calcium atoms are placed in the Ca-II site. Although one hydroxyl ion, three Ca-II, and three phosphates positions are at each corner of the unit cell, only 1/4 of them belong to each corner. Therefore, one HAP unit cell consists of two hydroxyl ions, six Ca-II, and six phosphates at 0.25c and 0.75c, whereas there are four Ca-I at 0.0c and 0.5c [5, 21–23].

The essential feature of HAP is the hexagonal framework of calcium atoms and phosphate groups surrounding a column of hydroxyl groups. From a crystallographic point of view, the arrangement of calcium atoms, phosphate, and hydroxyl groups in the crystal can be modeled as in **Figure 9** [24, 25]. Within the atomic lattices of HAP, two distinct unconnected channels can be delineated: a small channel and a large

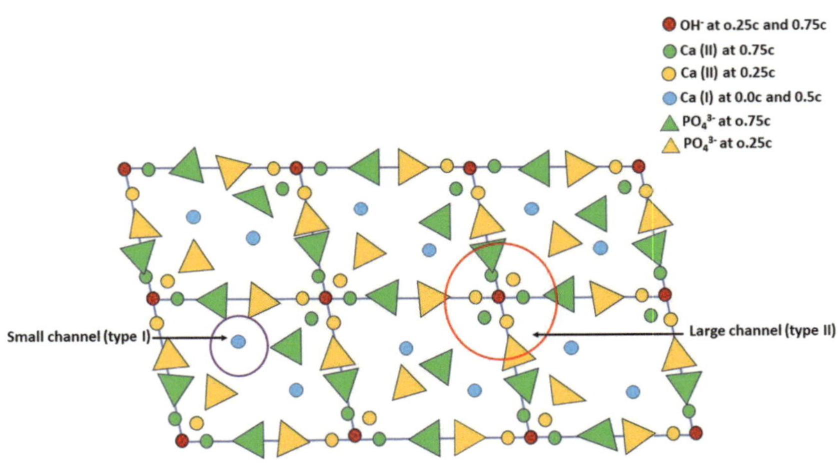


**Figure 10.**
*Schematic picture of the two channels of HAP unit cells. The projection of the structure $Ca_4(1)Ca_6(II)(PO_4)_6(OH)_2$ along the c-axis. In this atomic lattice, small (type I) and large (type II) channels can be described (Adapted from Ref. [26]) (see in-text explanations for details).*

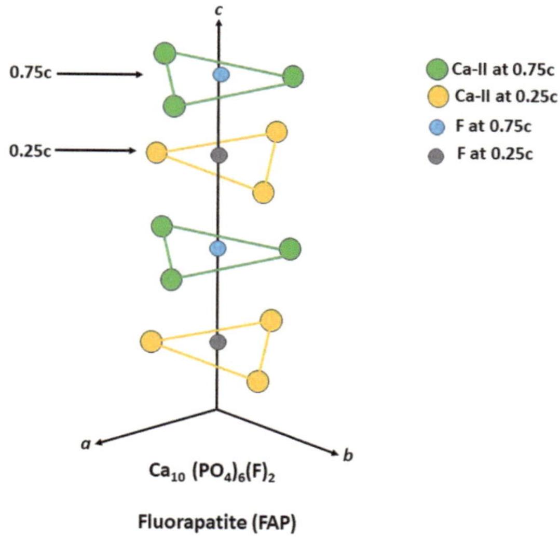


**Figure 11.**
*A view of fluorapatite (FAP) projecting perpendicular to the c-axis. In the central c-axis, there is a substitution of the hydroxyl ion by a fluoride ion. Fluoride ions replace hydroxyl ions on a 1:1 basis and are randomly dispersed along the c-axis. Calcium-II ions surround the screw axis at 0.25c and 0.75c. The fluoride ions are positioned within the triangular Ca-II configuration at 0.25c and 0.75c. It is important to note that this figure illustrates fluoride ions and Ca-II ions, with Ca-I ions and phosphates omitted for clarity.*

channel. The first channel (type I) possesses a diameter of 0.25 nm and is surrounded by Ca-I. This channel exhibits coordination 9 with the oxygen atoms of the phosphate tetrahedrons, resulting in the formation of a polyhedron. The second channel (type II) holds significance in the properties of HAP, featuring a larger diameter than the preceding one (ranging from 0.3 to 0.45 nm). It includes six additional Ca atoms, denoted as Ca-II, positioned at the periphery of the channel (**Figure 10**) [26, 27]. Various atom substitutions can take place in the large channel. For instance, hydroxyl groups can undergo substitution by anions such as fluoride (**Figure 11**), and phosphate groups can be substituted by other anions, such as carbonate [23, 28, 29].

## 3. Biological hydroxyapatites

Biologically, HAP in enamel is highly non-stoichiometric. The molar ratio of calcium to phosphorus in enamel ranged from 1.50 to 1.67, whereas the ratio in stoichiometric HAP remains constant at 1.67. The presence of non-stoichiometric HAP is due to the loss of $Ca^{2+}$ ions, resulting in an electrical imbalance that is rectified by the inclusion of $H^+$ ions and a reduction in $OH^-$ ions. This phenomenon is represented by the formula $Ca_{10-Z}(HPO_4)_Z(PO_4)_{6-Z}(OH)_{2-Z}$; where $0 < Z < 1$ [26, 30]. Consequently, enamel mineral differs from ideal HAP, incorporating ions such as $HPO_4^{2-}$, $CO_3^{2-}$, $Na^+$, $F^-$, and others into its apatite lattice. Within the HAP structure of enamel, the carbonate group occupies two distinct positions: the hydroxide position (A) and the phosphate position (B). Approximately 11 weight% of the total carbonate in deciduous enamel is situated in position A, while 10 weight% of the total carbonate in permanent enamel is found in the same position. Carbonates play a crucial role in enamel maturation and may contribute to the initial phase of dental caries formation [31].

## 4. Surface properties of enamel

The Stern-Gouy electrical double-layer theory is used to describe the microscopic structure at the solid surface [32]. The outer enamel layer (less than 1 μm from the anatomical surface) is most likely a non-stoichiometric apatite. The outer surface of enamel exhibits surface area fractions of calcium, phosphates, and hydroxyl ions about 16.5, 78.4, and 5.1%, respectively [33]. Phosphoric acid displays three pKa values (2.1, 7.2, and 12.7). While $PO_4^{3-}$, $HPO_4^{2-}$, $H_2PO^{4-}$, and $H_3PO_4$ can all be found in aqueous solutions, $HPO_4^{2-}$ (62%) and $H_2PO_4^{-}$ (38%) are predominantly present at neutral pH [34]. Consequently, the outer surface of enamel acquires a negative charge due to the presence of $HPO_4^{2-}$ and $H_2PO^{4-}$groups. This negative charge facilitates the formation of the Stern layer, also recognized as the calcium-rich layer, which firmly adheres to the enamel surfaces (**Figure 12**) [33, 35].

## 5. The oral environment

The tooth surface is continually immersed in either saliva or gingival crevicular fluid. Saliva plays an important role in maintaining enamel integrity by regulating the demineralization and remineralization of enamel minerals. The active concentrations of calcium, phosphate, and fluoride ions in saliva are key factors influencing the stability of enamel hydroxyapatite, along with salivary pH. Elevated concentrations of calcium and phosphate in saliva facilitate ionic exchanges directed toward the tooth surfaces, initiating post-eruptive maturation from the time of tooth eruption [36]. As soon as saliva contacts tooth surfaces, salivary glycoproteins selectively adsorb to the tooth surface to form an acquired salivary pellicle. The adsorbed salivary components

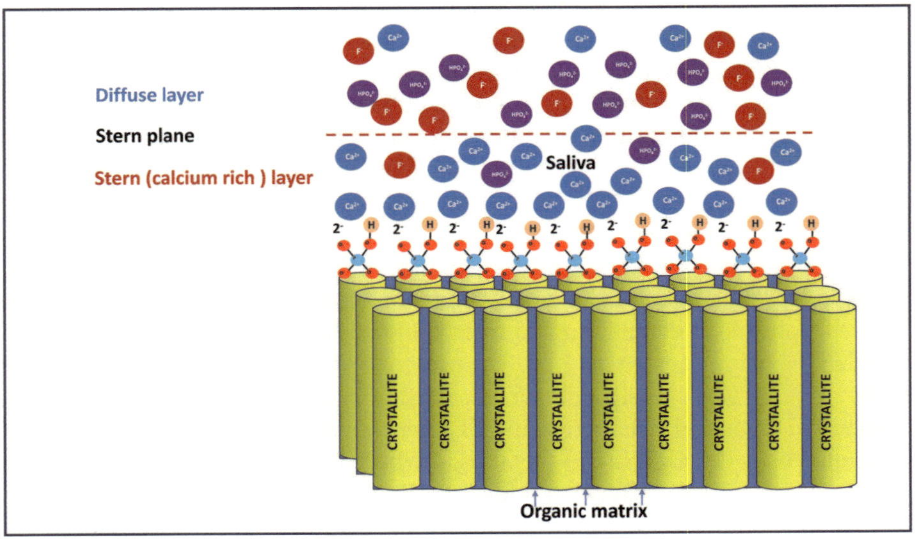


**Figure 12.**
*A schematic representation of the solid-liquid interface of enamel crystallites. Typically, solid enamel carries a negative charge attributed to the presence of $HPO_4^{2-}$. This negative charge results in the formation of the Stern layer, also known as the calcium-rich layer, which tightly adheres to the enamel surfaces. This layer is integral and inseparable from the enamel. In the solution phase, the remaining ions present in saliva, including calcium ions, acid phosphates, and fluorides, are dispersed by electrostatic interactions, forming what is known as the diffuse layer. The diffuse layer represents the distribution of these ions in the solution surrounding the enamel.*

not only sustain high levels of calcium and phosphate within saliva but also enhance the adherence of oral bacteria to tooth surfaces [37].

The mouth contains a wide range of microorganisms, which is more diverse than those found in other parts of the body. It is likely that the oral cavity offers various ecological niches [38]. Most oral bacteria are attached to the numerous surfaces in the oral cavity as oral biofilm (e.g., dental biofilm on tooth surfaces), where they are constantly bathed in either saliva or gingival crevicular fluid, providing hydration to the oral biofilm as well as nutrient to oral bacteria [39]. Dental biofilm contributes to the development of oral diseases such as dental caries and periodontal diseases. However, the consistent presence of fluoride ions in saliva and plaque fluids is crucial for protecting enamel from demineralization when facing caries threats [40]. Alongside the cariogenic environment, enamel can also be exposed to acidic conditions, particularly through the consumption of acidic foods and beverages. Dental wear, such as dental erosion, is frequently observed in individuals who regularly consume sports and/or soft drinks [41].

## 6. Acquired salivary pellicle formation, composition, and function

An acquired salivary pellicle forms when saliva comes into contact with the tooth [42]. This pellicle is comprised of proteins, lipids, carbohydrates, and other macromolecules. The components of the acquired salivary pellicle originate from various sources, including salivary gland secretion, gingival crevicular fluid, blood, products from the oral mucosa, oral bacteria, and diet [43]. Primarily, the acquired salivary pellicle is composed of adsorbed salivary proteins. Examples include albumin, amylase, carbonic anhydrase I-II, VI, cystatins, fibrinogen, fibronectin, histatins, immunoglobulins, lactoferrin, lysozyme, salivary mucins MG1 (MUC5B) and MG2 (MUC7), myeloperoxidase, proline-rich proteins (PRPs), secretory IgA, and statherin [44, 45]. Additional macromolecules in the acquired salivary pellicle include lipids and carbohydrates, encompassing glycolipids, phospholipids, and glycoproteins [43]. Importantly, the composition of the acquired salivary pellicle varies among individuals [46]. **Figure 13** shows the acquired salivary pellicle structure with the atomic force microscopy (AFM) technique [43, 47]. The acquired salivary pellicle forms by

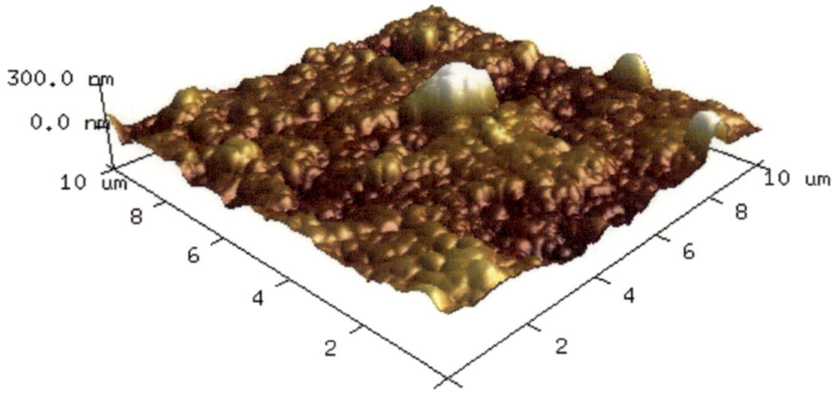


**Figure 13.**
*AFM image of the acquired pellicle structure. AFM image of in vitro acquired salivary pellicle morphology on enamel block after 2-h formation time. This view highlights the three-dimensional topographic differences as a result of the acquired pellicle layer adsorbed onto the enamel surface.*

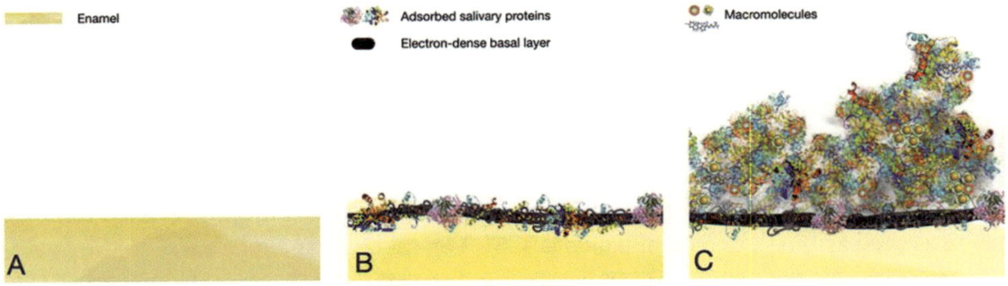


**Figure 14.**
*Schematic representation of pellicle formation. (A) Enamel surface, (B) electron-dense basal layer at initial stage: attachment of pellicle precursor proteins, (C) outer globular layer at maturation stage: equilibrium between adsorption and desorption of macromolecules. This image is adapted from a courtesy image by Chawhuaveang et al. [43].*

dynamic and selective processes of adsorbed and desorbed salivary proteins on the enamel surface [42]. Transmission electron micrography shows that the acquired salivary pellicle structure contains an electron-dense basal layer and an outer globular layer [43, 48].

The initial stage of acquired salivary pellicle occurs within seconds to a couple of minutes. The adsorbed salivary proteins attach to the enamel surface to form the electron-dense basal layer *via* electrostatic interactions [44, 49]. The electron-dense basal layer consists of a densely globular structure of phosphate and calcium-binding peptides, precursors of acquired salivary pellicle, and acid-resistance proteins [42, 50], such as PRPs, histatins, mucins, and statherin [51–53]. This layer is characterized by high acid resistance and strongly adheres to enamel crystals [45, 51]. The thickness of the electron-dense basal layer at the initial stage is approximately 10–20 nm [54]. It takes 60–120 minutes to reach the maturation stage and stays at a steady level for several hours [42, 54]. The thickness of the outer globular layer at the maturation stage is approximately 100–1000 nm [54]. The outer globular layer consists of other macromolecules and adsorbed proteins such as albumin, amylase, carbonic anhydrase, and mucins [45, 50]. This outer globular layer is composed of different sizes of micelle-like globular and granular structures. It exhibits knotted structures and globular-like structure [42, 55]. The formation mechanism of the acquired pellicle is shown in **Figure 14** [43]. The functions of the acquired salivary pellicle have been approved for determining the primary colonizers of oral bacteria [56], lubricating the tooth surface during mastication and speech [43], maintaining mineral homeostasis [47], and protecting the tooth surface against dental caries and dental erosion [49, 53].

## 7. Dental biofilm (dental plaque)

### 7.1 Dental biofilm formation

As mentioned above, the enamel surfaces of teeth are generally covered by the acquired salivary pellicle, which is essentially free of bacteria. Following tooth cleaning, some bacteria attach to the pellicle shortly afterward. While remnants of dental biofilm left due to incomplete removal by oral hygiene procedures may account for some bacteria, the majority of newly deposited bacteria come directly from oral fluids [57].

Biofilm is a microbial community embedded in a matrix and attached to different surfaces or environments. Bacteria form biofilms in every substratum and their associated infections in plants, animals, and humans [58]. In human body, bacterial biofilms can attach to various clinical devices and microflora-exposed tissues including tooth surfaces [58, 59]. Biofilms offer a habitat for bacteria and prevent them from pH varying and nutrient deficiency. Bacteria in a biofilm are more resistant to antibacterial or chemical treatments compared with that of planktonic bacteria [60].

The term "dental plaque" was probably first described by G.V. Black in 1886 when he collected a group of microorganisms on early carious lesions. Therefore, dental plaque is the biofilm on the tooth surface. Dental biofilms have common properties, that is, the presence of an extracellular polysaccharide substances (EPS) matrix and drug resistance [61]. The dental biofilm has advantages over the planktonic bacteria in saliva in terms of preventing elimination from rinsing or swallowing, defending against pathogen invasion and host mediators. Oral biofilms are classified by the composition and differ at distinct locations, including (1) supragingival biofilm and (2) subgingival biofilm. The supragingival biofilm is located on tooth surfaces, mostly contains Gram-positive and facultatively anaerobic bacteria (especially *Streptococcus* spp.), and is associated with dental caries. In contrast, the subgingival biofilm is located in gingival crevice, mostly contains Gram-negative and obligately anaerobic bacteria, that is, *Porphyromonas gingivalis,* and correlates with periodontitis [59].

Dental biofilm formation occurs within a few hours in a sequential event consisting of four stages (**Figure 15**): (1) initial colonization of tooth surfaces covered with an acquired salivary pellicle, (2) rapid bacterial growth and EPS production, (3) bacterial coadhesion and coaggregation, and (4) maturation and dispersion [62]. At stage 1, the tooth surfaces exposed to the oral environment are steadily covered by a conditioning film or acquired salivary pellicle, which is mostly derived from the adsorption of

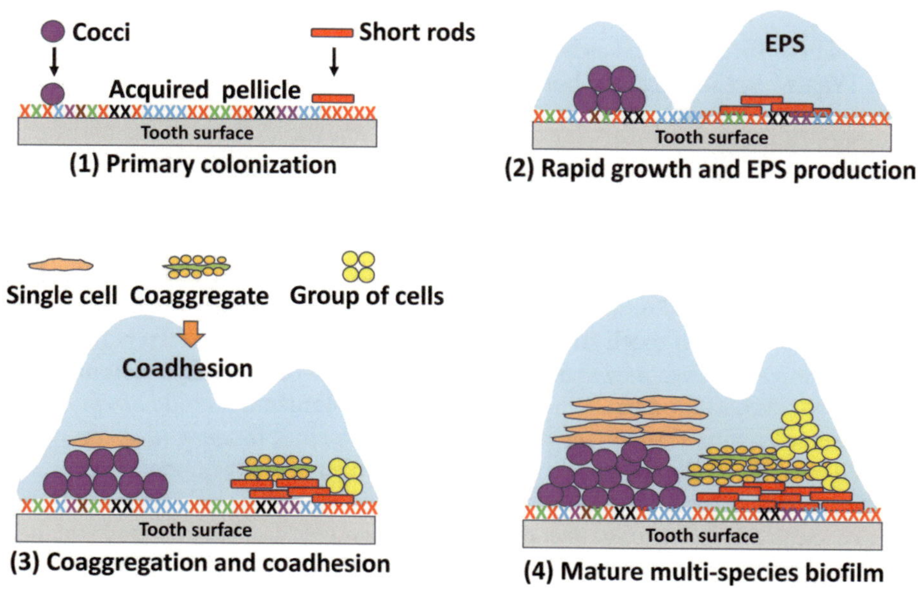


**Figure 15.**
*Dental biofilm formation. (1) primary colonizers adhere to a tooth surface covered with acquired salivary pellicle; (2) rapid cell growth, division, and production of EPS resulting in microcolony formation; (3) coadhesion of single bacterial cell, coaggregated bacteria, and groups of identical bacteria into the young multispecies dental biofilm; and (4) maturation and the development of clonal mosaics within the multispecies dental biofilm.*

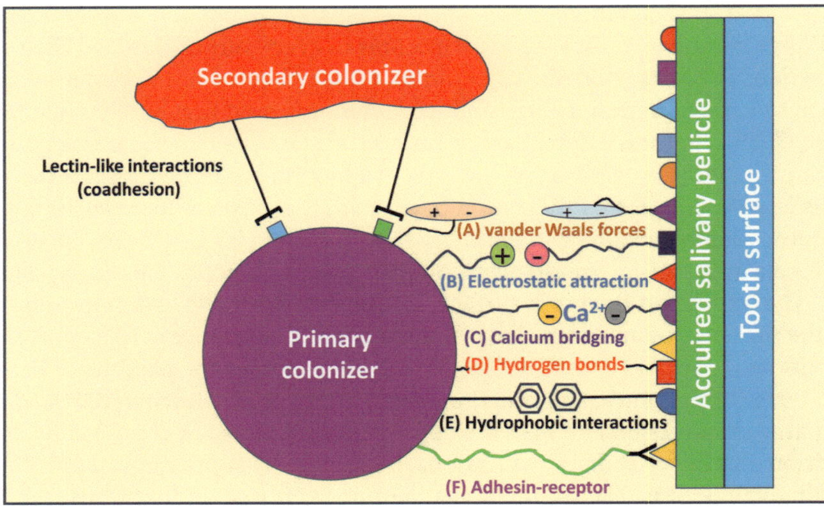


**Figure 16.**
*Schematic representation of initial bacterial adherence to tooth surfaces. Initial bacterial approach and adhesion to a pellicle-coated tooth surface are mediated by (A) van der Waals forces, (B) electrostatic attraction, (C) calcium bridging, (D) hydrogen bond, (E) hydrophobic interactions, and (F) adhesion-receptor interactions. Notably, the primary colonizers provided new specific receptors for the coadhesion of secondary colonizers.*

organic and inorganic molecules in saliva. Some proteins in the pellicle offer binding sites for adhesion of the planktonic initial bacteria, mainly from the genera *Streptococcus* and *Actinomyces* [63]. The first attachment of bacteria to the tooth surface covered by the pellicle is facilitated by fimbriae, as well as by various forces at different ranges, resulting in specific interactions between receptors and adhesins. These forces can be either attractive (involving hydrophobic interactions, van der Waals forces, hydrogen bonds, and calcium bridges), repulsive (involving electrostatic interactions), or a combination of both (involving acid-base interactions) (**Figure 16**) [64, 65].

Initially, dental biofilm forms through the interactions of both adhered and planktonic bacteria, with its further maturation being dominated by the proliferation and differentiation of the adhered bacteria [66]. The bacterial adhesion to an acquired salivary pellicle represents one of the most important factors in the bacterial colonization of tooth surfaces. Some bacteria, known as early or primary colonizers, are capable of colonizing on tooth surfaces coated by the acquired salivary pellicle. The primary colonizers create new specific receptors for late or secondary colonizers that are unable to directly bind to the pellicle. The early colonizers include *Streptococci* spp., *Actinomyces* spp., *Capnocytophaga* spp., *Eikenella* spp., *Haemophilus* spp., and *Veillonella* spp. However, 60–80% of primary colonizers are streptococci. Then, the early adherent streptococci on tooth surfaces recruit secondary colonizers to form a biofilm through an autoaggregation or coaggregation process. Subsequent attached bacterial species include *Fusobacterium nucleatum*, *Treponema* spp., *Porphylomonas gingivalis*, and *Aggregatibacter actinomycetemcomitans* (**Figure 17**) [67–69].

In Stage 2, after the initial bacteria have been successfully colonized, they consequently enter a logarithmic growth phase, and the biofilm will start differentiating as a highly structured community. Interspecies communication occurs by using the quorum-sensing system. This system facilitates biofilm differentiation, bacterial

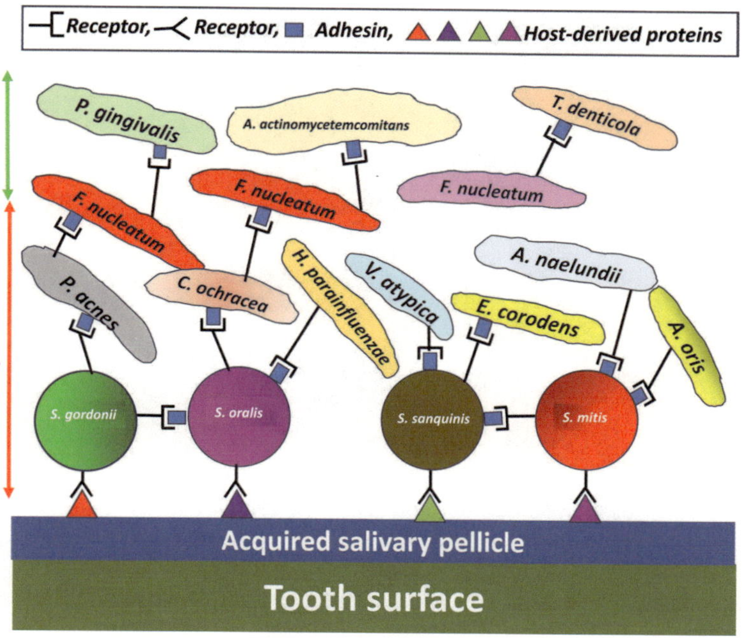


**Figure 17.**
*Schematic representation of oral bacterial colonization. Bacterial colonization starts with the adhesion of early colonizers (such as* Streptococci *spp.,* Actinomyces *spp.,* Capnocytophaga *spp.,* Eikenella *spp.,* Haemophilus *spp., and* Veillonella *spp.) to host-derived proteins in acquired salivary pellicle. Consequently, the early colonizers recruit other oral bacteria to produce late colonizers. The late colonizers include* Fusobacterium nucleatum, Treponema *spp.,* Porphylomonas gingivalis, *and* Aggregatibacter actinomycetemcomitans *(Adapted from Ref. [67]).*

metabolism, EPS production, and biofilm maturation (**Figure 18**) [68, 70]. In Stage 3, the growth of early colonizers on the dental surface introduces new binding sites for other species. This binding process fosters coadhesion and coaggregation, leading to the formation of a multi-species biofilm (**Figure 19**) [71]. In Stage 4, synergistic and antagonistic interactions within the biofilm contribute to food and oxygen exchange. This exchange strengthens the biofilm matrix, facilitates equilibrated homeostasis, and culminates in the maturation of the biofilm. Eventually, bacteria are released from the matured biofilm, undergoing reorganization on other surfaces [63].

Drug resistance is one of the effective synergistic interactions within dental biofilm. Chlorhexidine is a common antiseptic mouthwash used for dental plaque controlling [72]. An *in vitro* study using live/dead staining and confocal laser scanning microscopy demonstrated that chlorhexidine exhibits bactericidal penetration (red color) into dental biofilm surface (approximately 50% of total biofilm structure) (**Figure 20**). In contrast, the living bacteria (green color) were observed in the middle to bottom of the biofilm. This confirmed the resistant capability against chlorhexidine of some bacteria in dental plaque.

### 7.2 Sugar metabolism and acid production

Among dietary carbohydrates, sucrose can induce significant biochemical and physiological changes during dental biofilm formation, rendering it one of the most

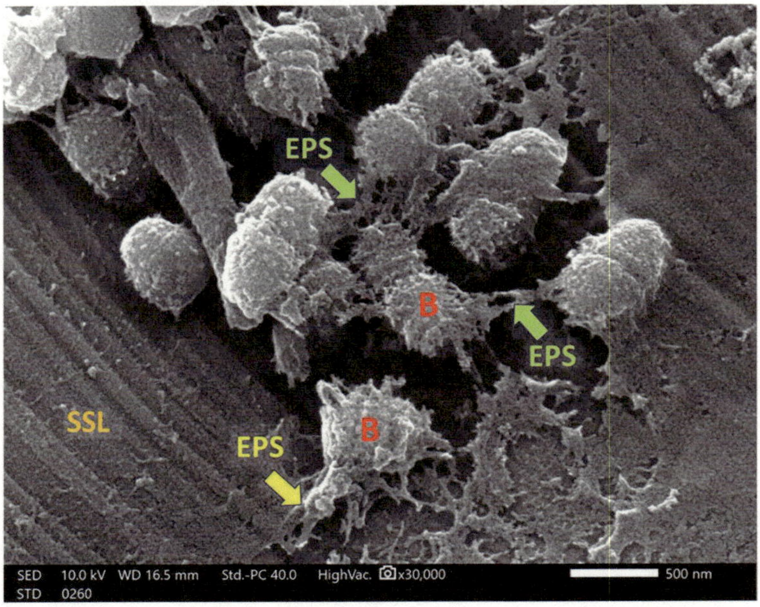


**Figure 18.**
*SEM of dental biofilm. Dental biofilm accumulated on the stainless steel ligature (SSL) after 6 weeks of permanence in the mouth of an orthodontic patient. Bacterial cells (B) firmly adhere to the SSL surface* via *EPS (yellow arrow). The EPS also mediated cell-cell (green arrow) accumulation in biofilm formation (original magnification x 30,000) (Figure courtesy of Drs. Thanakorn Saengphen and Apiwat Ridhabhaya, International College of Dentistry, Walailak University, Bangkok, Thailand).*

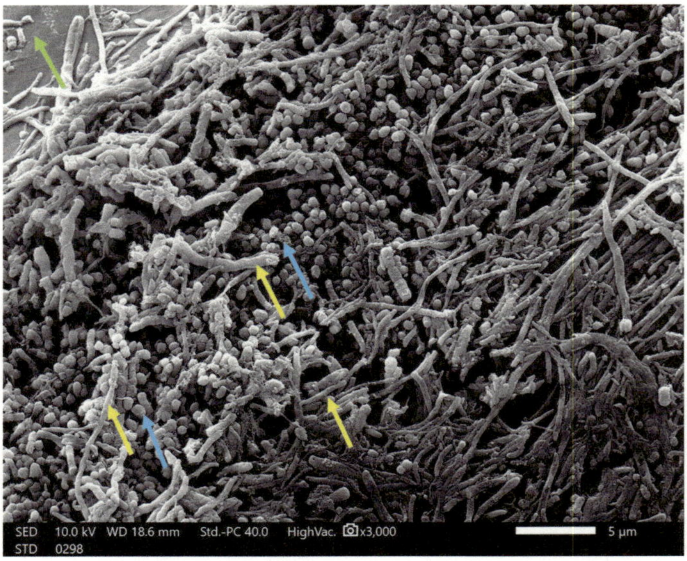


**Figure 19.**
*SEM micrograph of matured dental plaque. Plaque was developed on the SSL (green arrow) after 6 weeks of permanence in the mouth of an orthodontic patient. Mass of biofilm comprised of aggregated coccoid (blue arrow) intertwining with rod- and filament-shaped bacteria (yellow arrow) (original magnification X 3000) (Figure courtesy of Drs. Thanakorn Saengphen and Apiwat Ridhabhaya, International College of Dentistry, Walailak University, Bangkok, Thailand).*

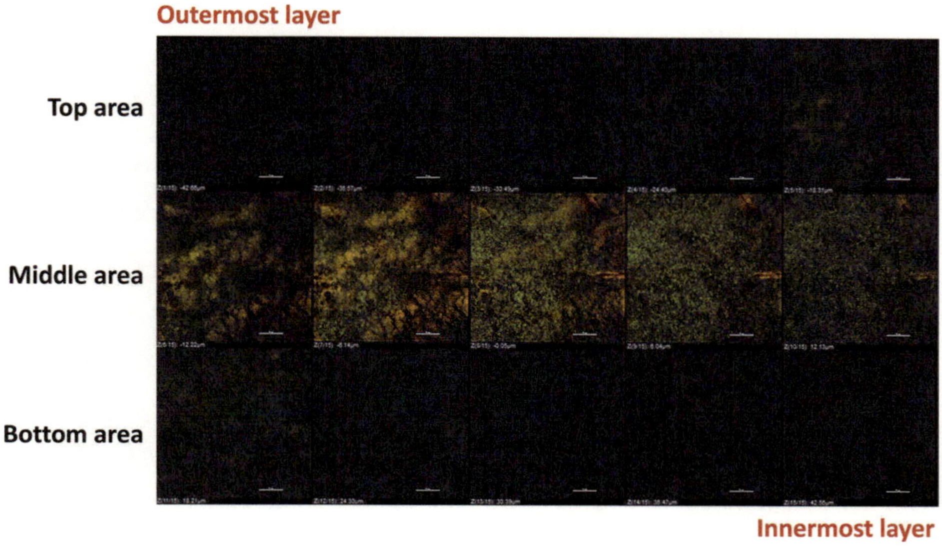


**Figure 20.**
*In vitro effects of chlorhexidine on bacterial biofilm. In vitro S. mutans biofilm is developed on a saliva-coated HAP surface and incubated for 48 h. Chlorhexidine (1 µg/ml) is used to treat the biofilm. Live or dead bacteria are studied using Live/Dead® bacterial BacLight™ Bacterial Viability Kit (Invitrogen Molecular Probes, Carlsbad, CA, USA). Live and dead bacteria are stained by SYTO 9—green fluorescent and propidium iodide—red fluorescent, respectively. The stained biofilm is scanned and visualized from top to bottom (each layer thickness is approximately 5 µm) using confocal laser scanning microscope (EclipseTi; Nikon Instrument Inc., Tokyo, Japan).*

cariogenic carbohydrates. The glycolysis pathway metabolizes sucrose to acids, with lactic acid produced at high sugar concentrations and acetic acid, formic acid, and ethanol generated at low sugar concentrations. Energy generated during glycolysis is essential for bacterial growth. Sucrose also functions as a substrate for the synthesis of intracellular polysaccharides (IPS) and EPS in dental biofilms. IPS can be catabolized to acids in the absence of dietary sugars. EPS plays a crucial role in dental biofilm formation. It fosters the development of a matrix, improving bacterial attachment and the subsequent buildup of bacteria within dental biofilms. Moreover, it contributes to the structural strength and volume of dental biofilms, heightening the acidity of the dental biofilm matrix [66, 73–75].

The dental biofilm maintains homeostasis to promote oral health, providing advantages to the normal flora and the host. In ordinary biofilm, *S. mitis*, *S. sanguinis*, and *S. cristatus* use arginine deiminase to suppress adhesion and the expression of virulent factors in *P. gingivalis* [76, 77]. In addition, *S. salivarius*, *S. mitis*, *S. gordonii*, *S. sanguinis*, *S. cristatus*, and *A. naeslundii* use salivary lactoperoxidase system to buffer the acid produced by certain cariogenic bacteria. The lactoperoxidase system also increases $H_2O_2$, which is toxic to *S. mutans*. This evidence confirms that bacterial interaction promotes biofilm neutralization and maintains the demineralization/remineralization balance to prevent dental caries [77, 78].

The "Ecological plaque hypothesis" (EPH) has clearly explained ecological shift from normal dental plaque forward to caries risk plaque [79]. When there is a high frequent consumption of carbohydrates and fermentable sugars, most of the bacteria ferment the sugar and produce the acids as by-products. This decreases the pH in the dental biofilm from relatively neutral conditions (pH 6.0–7.0) to a more acidic pH (5.5),

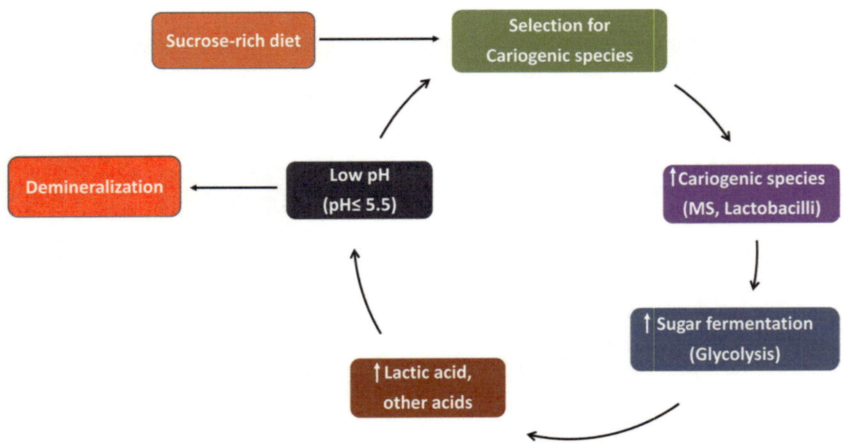


**Figure 21.**
*EPH and caries. The diagram depicts the dynamic relationship that exists between the dental plaque and the local environment, according to EPH (Adapted from Ref. [81]).*

which reduces the buffering capacity of saliva [80]. The acidic environment favors the rapid growth of cariogenic bacteria including mutans streptococci (MS), *Actinomyces*, and *Lactobacillus*. MS, especially *S. mutans,* has relatively high acidogenic potential compared with the non-mutans group in terms of sugar uptake and metabolism. The cariogenic bacteria ferment carbohydrates by degrading glucose into pyruvate and lactate/acetate/formate, creating the cariogenic environment (**Figure 21**) [81, 82].

Based on EPH, a disclosing staining agent has been developed to assess caries risk in patient's dental biofilm. Currently, the 3-tone staining gel (GC Tri-plaque ID Gel™, GC Corporation, Japan) is one of the practical tools used for evaluating status and

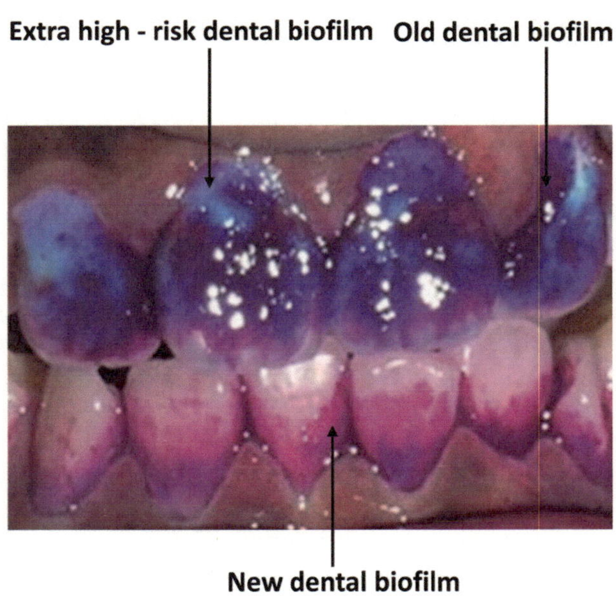


**Figure 22.**
*Dental biofilm staining with GC Tri-plaque ID Gel$^{TM}$. Dental biofilm is stained according to the company's instructions. The result is shown in three colors based on the dental biofilm conditions: new dental biofilm (pink), old dental biofilm (blue/purple), and extra high-risk dental biofilm (light blue).*

acidic change in dental biofilm. The gel contains sucrose and pigments (blue and red) that can penetrate and stain the dental biofilm, resulting in three colors based on the dental biofilm status. The pink color indicates newly formed dental biofilm in its initiation stage without EPS. Meanwhile, blue/purple blues represent old dental biofilm, with light blue denoting extra high-risk or cariogenic dental biofilm (**Figure 22**) [83]. The environmental change in dental biofilm due to high frequent sugar consumption provides an acidic environment and ecological shift to cariogenic bacteria accumulation, and disrupts the demineralization/remineralization balance in enamel and initiating carious lesions [79].

## 8. Demineralization and remineralization

Demineralization of HAP is initiated by protonated ions of phosphates ($PO_4^{3-}$ + $H^+$; $HPO_4^{2-}$) and hydroxyl groups ($OH^-$ + $H^+$; $H_2O$) in the apatite lattices. According to Coulomb's law, calcium ions in HAP will therefore not be bound to an adequate extent but rather will be lost. It is worth noting that the attractive forces between ions in water are significantly weaker, about 1/80th, compared to those in a vacuum. As per Coulomb's law, this suggests that HAP is prone to dissolve in water [19]. As mentioned above, organic acids, especially lactic acid, are generated by cariogenic bacteria in dental biofilm, particularly, in the presence of high sugar concentrations. In theory, when the pH of dental biofilm decreases, there comes a point where enamel HAP starts to dissolve. This particular point is often termed as the critical pH. The physiological concentration of salivary calcium is about 1.0 mmol/L. This makes the critical pH, which is the tipping point between enamel de- and remineralization, to be about pH 5.5, that is for healthy resting adults producing normal saliva [19, 84, 85]. Notably, $PO_4^{3-}$ and $OH^-$ in the HAP are protonated by $H^+$ if the pH drops below critical pH (pH 5.5). Then, the phosphate and hydroxyl ions lose one negative charge, which is important for binding calcium ions. This causes a loss of minerals from the apatite lattices (**Figure 23**) [20].

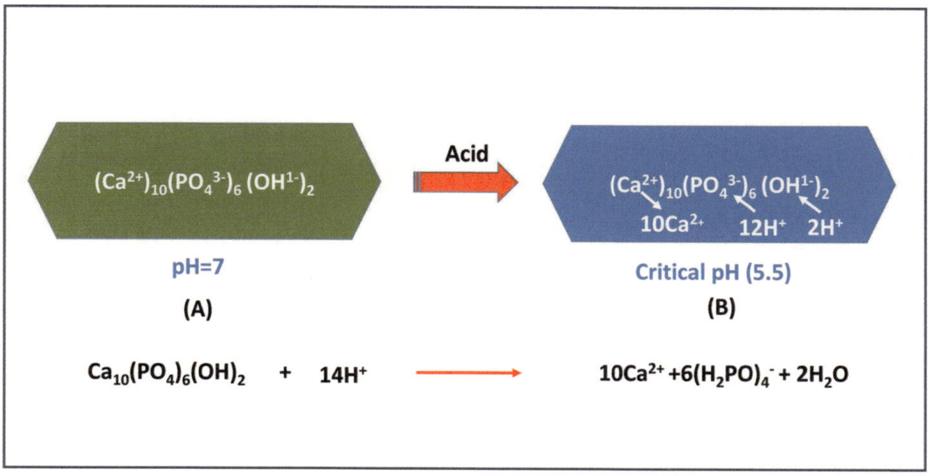


**Figure 23.**
*Schematic representation of HAP dissolution in the acid environment. (A) HAP is stable at pH 7. (B) The $PO_4^{3-}$ and $OH^-$ ions from the HAP are protonated by $H^+$ ions if the pH drops below critical pH (pH 5.5). Then, the phosphate and hydroxyl ions lose one negative charge, which is important to bind $Ca^{2+}$. This causes a loss of minerals from the HAP lattices (Adapted from Ref. [20]).*

In essence, ionic solids, such as HAP, undergo constant reactions with the surrounding media. All minerals exhibit an inherent and fixed solubility in water at any given temperature. Water molecules are essential in removing ions from the crystal surface by diminishing the electrostatic interactions between positively and negatively charged ions, which is facilitated by water's high dielectric constant. Additionally, water molecules create hydration shells around the ions that are released. The energy of these hydration shells exceeds the lattice energy holding the crystal together [86]. When an ionic solid (s) is in water, it will release an equal number of constituent ions into the aqueous (aq) solution at equilibrium. When solid HAP is dissolved in a solution, it breaks down into $Ca^{2+}$, ${PO_4}^{3-}$, and $OH^-$ as follows:

$$Ca_{10}(PO_4)_6(OH)_2\ (s)\ \leftrightarrow\ 10Ca^{2+}\ (aq) + 6\ (PO_4)^{3-}\ (aq) + 2OH^-\ (aq).$$

This type of chemical equilibrium is described by the solubility product constant (Ksp). The Ksp of HAP is simply expressed to:

$$Ksp = \left[Ca^{2+}\right]^{10} x \left[{PO_4}^{3-}\right]^{6} x [OH^-]^2 \text{ or } \left[Ca^{2+}\right]^{5} x \left[{PO_4}^{3-}\right]^{3} x [OH^-].$$

It should be noted that the Ksp for a particular crystal is approximated to be a constant that is characteristic of that crystal. A crystal with a low Ksp is less soluble than a high Ksp. For example, the Ksp for HAP $[Ca_{10}(PO_4)_6(OH)_2]$ is approximately $5.5x10^{-118}$ $(mol.L^{-1})^9$. HAP has a low Ksp because of the near close-packed structure, which minimizes the distance of charge separation in Coulomb's law. The Ksp for FAP $[Ca_{10}(PO_4)_6F_2]$ is about $5.0x10^{-123}$ $(mol.L^{-1})^9$. This indicates the comparatively

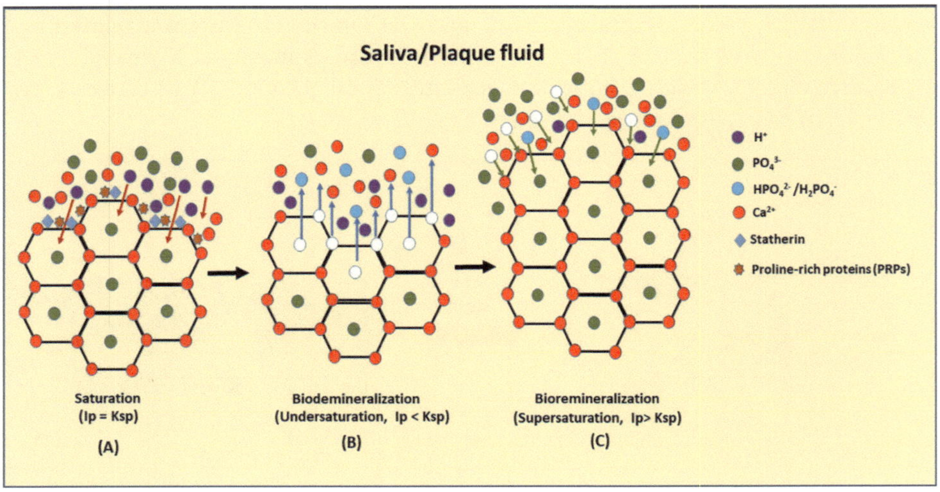


**Figure 24.**
*Schematic representation of biodemineralization and bioremineralization of enamel. (A) Chemical reaction conditions corresponding to saturation (Ip=Ksp) of enamel coated with statherin and PRPs result in the equilibrium between HAP degradation and formation. (B) Biodemineralization of enamel due to acidic where Ip is less than Ksp. When the pH decreases, hydrogen ions from the acid bind with the negative phosphate and hydroxyl ions from the acquired salivary pellicle and plaque fluids. Consequently, the Ip in the pellicle layer becomes unsaturated, causing a shift that favors demineralization. This results in the loss of calcium and phosphate ions from the crystal until a solubility equilibrium is reached. (C) If the concentration of protons adjacent to the enamel surface decreases and/or the concentration of calcium and phosphate ions increases, the Ip of the surrounding solution will be greater than Ksp for HAP. This results in a supersaturated condition that resists biodemineralization and favors biomineralization of enamel.*

denser arrangement of ions within the lattice and the slightly smaller size of unit cells in FAP when compared to HAP [19].

In various solutions like saliva, dental biofilm, or soft drinks, the ion activity product (Ip) associated with HAP is calculated using the same formula as Ksp, but with concentrations of reactants and products taken from any specific point in the reaction, not solely at the equilibrium point. When Ip equals Ksp, the solution is saturated with respect to HAP. If Ip is lower than Ksp, the solution is unsaturated. Conversely, if Ip exceeds Ksp, the solution is supersaturated [87]. It should be noted that, basically, human salivary calcium and phosphate ions are supersaturated with respect to HAP. However, spontaneous precipitation of HAP does not occur under physiological conditions. This phenomenon has been attributed to the inhibitory activities of statherin and the acidic proline-rich phosphoproteins (PRPs) in acquired salivary pellicle [88, 89]. Notably, salivary proteins, particularly statherin, act like a "negative" catalyst, or inhibitor, to slow down the process of demineralization. It has been reported that this can be by up to 50%. This occurs when the proteins modify the chemistry of the dissolution process at the enamel surface (**Figure 24**) [84].

## 9. Enamel dissolution in the cariogenic environment

HAP dissolution increases about 10-fold for a change of 1 pH unit [87]. Two reasons account for the heightened solubility of HAP when subjected to acid attack. Initially, $H^+$ ions resulting from the metabolic activity of cariogenic biofilms will combine with $OH^-$ ions encircling HAP, particularly within plaque fluids, resulting in the formation of $H_2O$ molecules. For example, if the pH of the aqueous solution drops from 7 to 5, the hydrogen ions will increase to $10^{-5}$ M, and $OH^-$ falls to $10^{-9}$ M, or to 1% of its previous concentration. Second, the proportions of the four phosphate species ($H_3PO_4$, $H_2PO_4^-$, $HPO_4^{2-}$, and $PO_4^{3-}$) in plaque fluid and saliva vary with pH, although the total phosphate concentration is $5 \times 10^{-3}$ mol/L, as is typical of saliva. The $H^+$ ions protonated $PO_4^{3-}$ in the plaque fluid to $HPO_4^{2-}$ and $H_2PO_4^-$. Therefore, as the pH of the plaque decreases, the concentration of $PO_4^{3-}$ in the fluid, and potentially in saliva, decreases as well. With both $PO_4^{3-}$ and $OH^-$ concentrations in plaque fluid diminishing at lower pH levels, it is anticipated that both ions will dissolve out of the enamel HAP to maintain equilibrium in the surrounding liquid solutions. This process is geared toward preserving neutrality and ultimately results in the dissolution of calcium from enamel HAP. However, in a cariogenic environment, the concentration of calcium remains relatively unaffected initially. Conversely, the concentrations of both $OH^-$ and $PO_4^{3-}$ undergo significant reduction, leading to a decrease in Ip to a value below the Ksp [19, 86, 87, 90]. Subsequently, the decrease in ionic attraction between cations and anions due to acid attack, as previously mentioned [19, 20], along with a decrease in Ip of surrounding fluids, results in mineral loss from enamel [86, 87, 90].

In the process of tooth decay, there is a cycle of demineralization and remineralization. During demineralization, dissolved $Ca^{2+}$ and $HPO_4^{2-}$ move actively from the advancing lesion front to the outer enamel surface. This movement is facilitated by the Galvani potential, which is created by the inward diffusion of protons. Upon reaching the tooth surface, the demineralized calcium and phosphate ions may combine with available fluoride, resulting in the formation of a mineral-rich layer at the lesion surface (**Figure 25**) [91, 92]. When the cariogenic conditions in the dental plaque subside, typically when the plaque pH rises above the critical pH of approximately 5.5, the remineralization phase begins. Unlike during demineralization, there is no outward movement of minerals from inside the lesion due to the absence of Galvani potential. Instead, calcium and phosphate concentrations at the tooth surface are higher than those in the lesion. Consequently, both ions from enamel demineralization, plaque fluids, and saliva passively diffuse into the enamel through micropores of the intact surface layer and particularly, intercrystallic spaces of the lesion. It is worth noting that the most effective remineralization initially occurs at the lesion boundary and then progresses toward the tooth's surface (**Figure 26**) [91, 92].

It is essential to note that the demineralized lesion in the initial carious stage is considered reversible to a certain extent through remineralization. However,

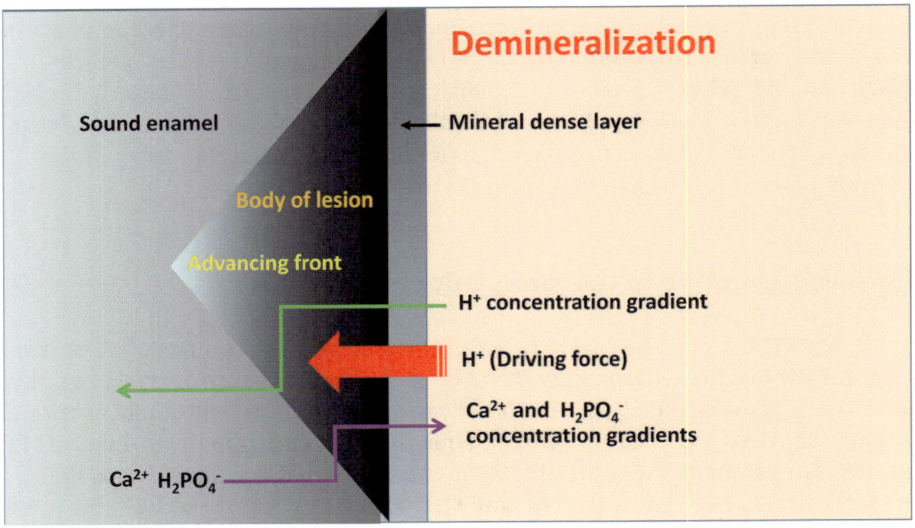


**Figure 25.**
*Schematic illustration of demineralization mechanism. An acid attack causes the Galvani potential, followed by active diffusion of calcium and phosphate ions out of the tooth (Modified from Ref. [91]).*

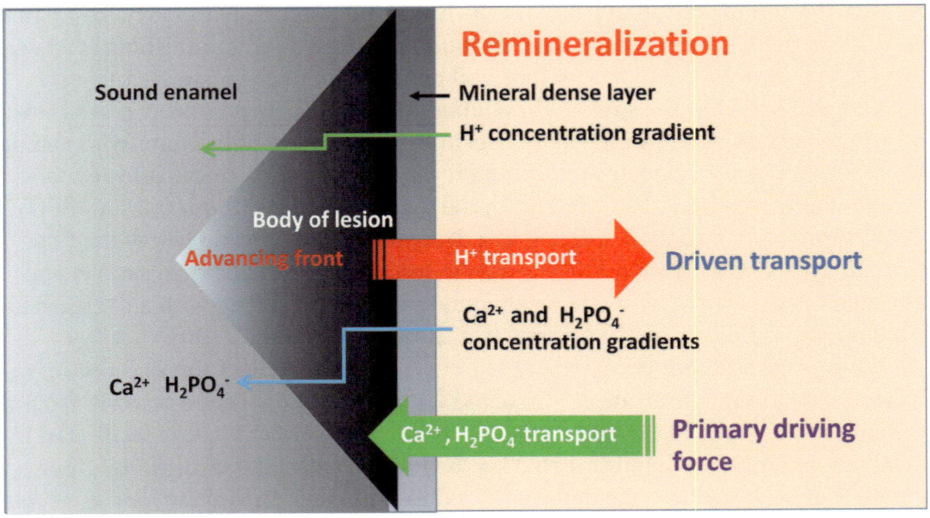


**Figure 26.**
*Schematic illustration of remineralization. Calcium and phosphate ions diffuse from a higher concentration outside of the tooth into the carious lesion, where precipitation occurs on existing apatite minerals at the lesion boundary, progressing to the enamel (Modified from Ref. [91]).*

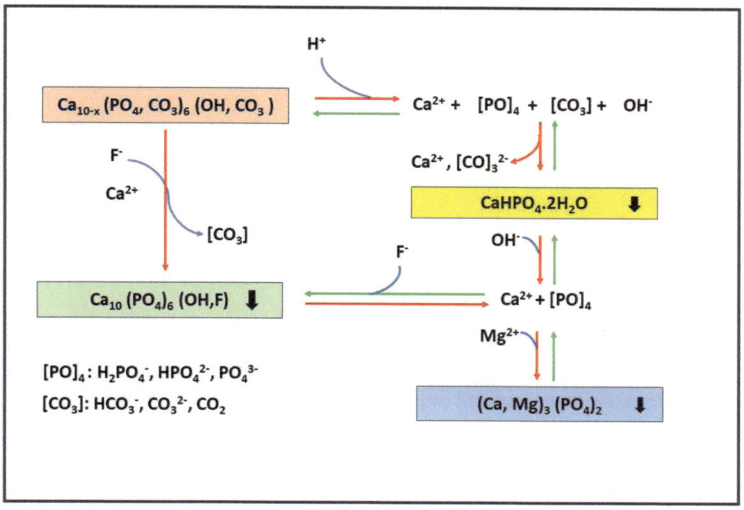


**Figure 27.**
*The postulated phase transition in the caries process. For the sake of simplicity, we here two assumptions: (i) the original tooth mineral is expressed as Ca-deficient apatites substituting carbonate at both $PO_4$ and OH lattice sites and (ii) the involvement of octacalcium phosphate [OCP, $Ca_8(HPO_4)_2(PO_4)_4{\cdot}5H_2O$] as an intermediate phase is excluded (Adapted from Ref. [93]).*

predominant demineralization leads to the formation of irreversible cavities. **Figure 27** outlines the hypothetical chain reactions occurring during demineralization/remineralization cycling. As demineralization initiates, a portion of the original tooth mineral dissolves, resulting in the formation of dicalcium phosphate dihydrate (DCPD, $CaHPO_4.2H_2O$) and octacalcium phosphate [OCP, $Ca_8(HPO_4)_2(PO_4)_4{\cdot}5H_2O$] under acidic conditions. When the acidogenic attack has subsided, and a neutral pH is returned, both DCPD and OCP may form apatite or carbonated hydroxyapatite [93, 94].

## 10. Initial caries

The first noticeable indication of enamel demineralization is the emergence of a white spot lesion (WSL). These lesions have a chalky white appearance, attributed to the increased porosity in the subsurface zone resulting from demineralization (**Figure 28**). The entrapment of air or saliva within the pores of demineralized enamel impacts light transmission due to variations in the refractive indices among enamel, air, and saliva [95, 96]. In the routine oral environment, demineralization and remineralization are dynamic processes that occur frequently, influencing the development or reversal of carious lesions. Analysis through scanning microradiography of naturally occurring initial carious enamel has revealed an average reduction of 30% mineral mass in the subsurface lesion [97, 98]. Examinations of initial carious lesions using various imbibition solvents and a polarized light microscope have identified four distinct zones: a relatively intact surface layer, the lesion body, a dark zone, and a translucent zone signifying the advancing front of the lesion (**Figure 29**) [99].

The transparent zone marks the innermost section of the advancing lesion front and shows minimal impact from caries attack. It demonstrates a pore volume ranging from 1 to 5%, indicating a slightly higher pore density compared to sound enamel, which generally maintains a pore volume of about 0.1%. Adjacent to the transparent

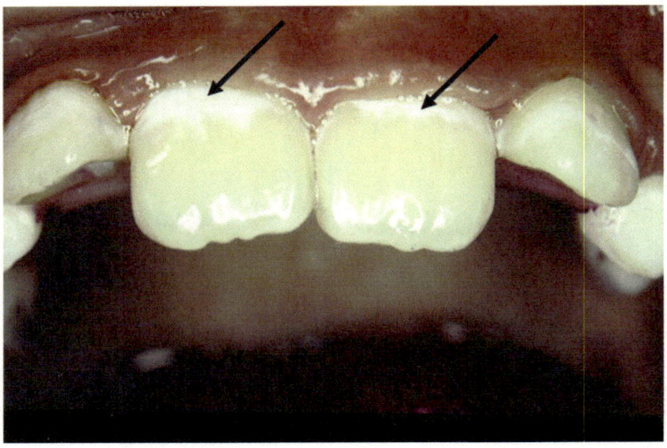

**Figure 28.**
*A clinical photograph of WSLs. WSLs (black arrows) are located at the incisor cervical regions. They are chalky white in appearance and feel slightly rough upon gentle probing.*

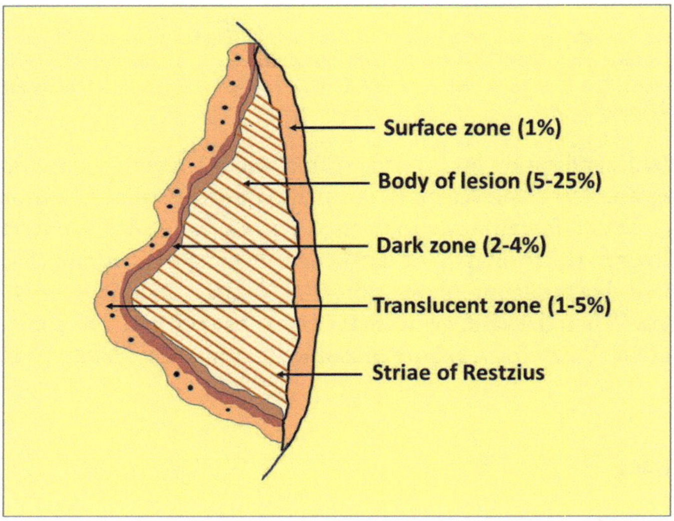


**Figure 29.**
*Diagram of histological changes and the pore volume distribution (%) in initial caries. The surface layer is due to mineral re-precipitations. In the subsurface, the body of the lesion is triangular in shape, with a summit oriented toward the DEJ. The striae of Retzius are well-marked in the body of lesion. The subsurface lesion displays two borders: one dark zone that is in progress and a reaction zone (limiting or translucent zone).*

zone is the dark zone, which, according to polarized light studies, displays a pore volume ranging from 2 to 4%. Sitting between the dark zone and the relatively unaffected surface layer, the body of the lesion represents the largest segment of initial carious enamel. This region undergoes the most significant demineralization, with a pore volume ranging from 5 to 25%. Notably, the striae of Retzius are prominently visible in this area, suggesting demineralization preferentially occurs in regions with higher porosity. The outermost "unaltered" surface remains relatively unaffected by the caries attack. It exhibits a slightly elevated pore volume (1%) compared to normal enamel [98, 100].

It is important to recognize that the development of enamel caries does not necessarily start with subsurface issues. Processes involving dissolution, precipitation, and protection from adsorbed proteins in an acquired salivary pellicle contribute to understanding the formation of porosity or solubility gradients. A white spot lesion typically signifies demineralization beneath the surface with heightened enamel porosity and porous outer tissues. Nonetheless, certain proteins like PRPs and others with protective properties can shield the surface from further demineralization and hinder crystal growth. Initially, due to their size, adsorbed proteins can penetrate and diffuse only into the deeper enamel layers at an intermediate stage of caries progression. Yet, as caries advance and pore sizes increase, smaller pellicle precursor and acid-resistant proteins may also infiltrate the subsurface lesion. Consequently, salivary proteins of varying sizes remain at different levels within the lesion, forming a protective coating during the demineralization process [101].

Scanning electron microscopy of the outer surface of initial caries showed two main structural features, accentuation of the perikymata and deep focal holes (**Figures 30** and **31**) [102–104]. Broadening of interprismatic spaces was commonly observed in affected areas. Mineral dissolution of prism cores was markedly observed when compared to that of prism borders (**Figure 32**). Demineralization of enamel shows loosely packed globular crystals with a few areas of the residual healthy enamel. These non-affected areas show no globular crystals (**Figure 33**) [104].

## 11. The interaction between enamel and fluoride in the oral environment

### 11.1 Formation of fluorapatite and calcium fluoride

Most toothpaste products available in stores typically contain 1000–1500 ppmF, typically as sodium fluoride (NaF) or sodium monofluorophosphate (MFP) [105]. Generally, the concentration of fluoride in the saliva is around 0.01 ppmF [106]. After using a fluoride product, the remaining fluoride in the mouth gets diluted by saliva. Salivary fluoride is distributed across various compartments in the oral cavity. Fluoride ions can be found in both saliva and dental plaque fluid. Fluorides in bound forms

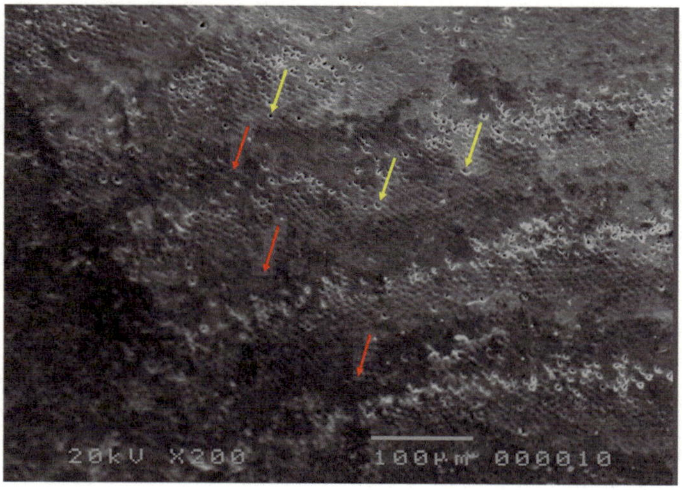


**Figure 30.**
*SEM of WSLs. Perikymata (red arrows): are prominent. The borders of the perikymata are flattened with an irregular shelf-like border. There are numerous deep focal holes (yellow arrows) (original magnification x 200; bar = 100 µm).*

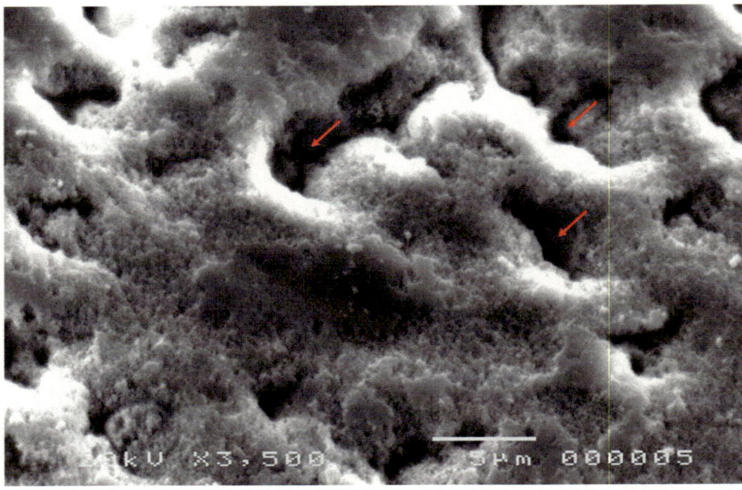


**Figure 31.**
*SEM of focal holes. Deep funnel-shaped focal holes (red arrows) were observed in the enamel surface of definite WSLs (original magnification x 3500; bar = 5 μm).*

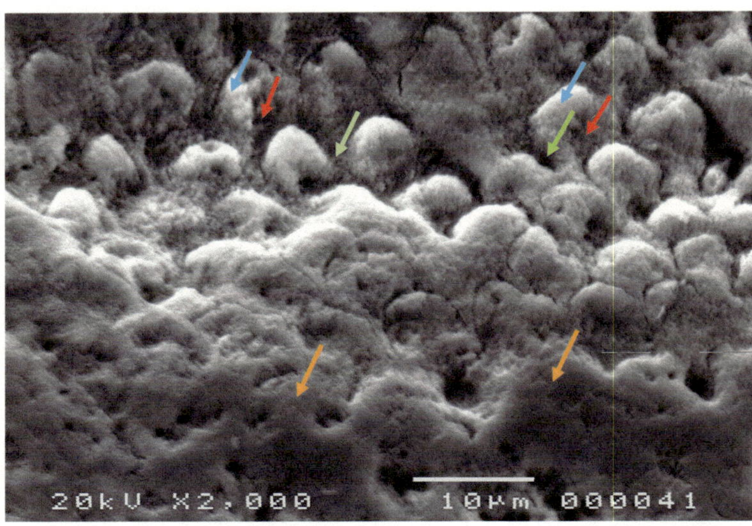


**Figure 32.**
*SEM of affected and unaffected areas. Broadening of interprismatic spaces (green arrows) was commonly observed in demineralized areas. Mineral dissolution is more advanced in prism cores (red arrows) compared to prism borders (blue arrows). Apparently, the intact areas (orange arrow) show relatively smooth surfaces (original magnification x 2000; bar = 10 μm).*

are present in dental plaque, calcium fluoride, enamel, and oral mucosa. Importantly, fluorides adsorbed onto the oral mucosal surface act as a significant reservoir for the slow release of fluoride. Fluoride that is swallowed is partially deposited in bones; however, it is not released back into the oral cavity (**Figure 34**) [107].

Fluoride presented in the oral fluid could interact with enamel HAP as follows [108]:

1. Ionic exchange reaction between F and OH in HAP

$$Ca_{10}(PO_4)_6(OH)_2 + 2F^- \rightarrow Ca_{10}(PO_4)_6F_2 + 2OH^- \quad (1)$$

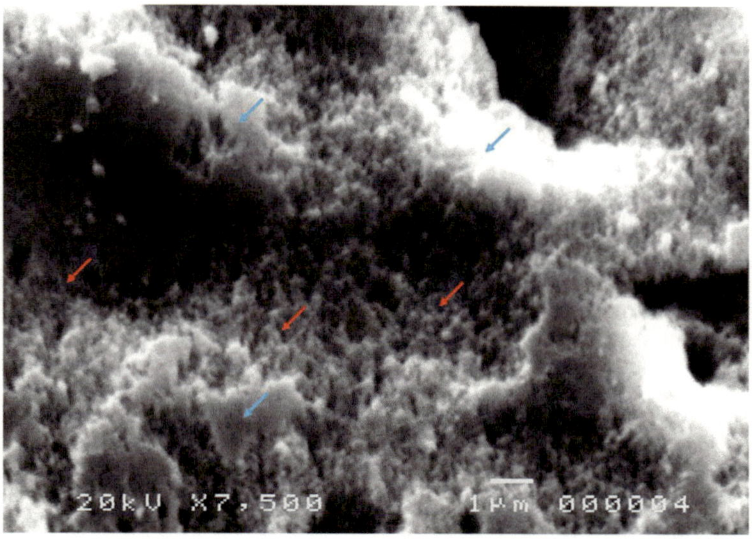


**Figure 33.**
*SEM of demineralized crystals. At higher magnification (x 7500; bar = 1 µm), the lesional surface shows loosely packed globular crystals (red arrows) with a few areas of the residual smooth enamel surface (blue arrows) of non-affected enamel. These non-affected areas show no globular crystals.*

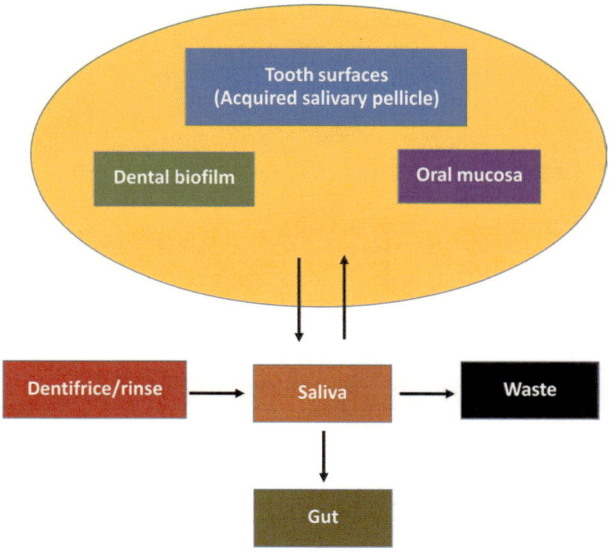


**Figure 34.**
*The fate of fluoride after using a fluoride product. Fluoride in saliva is exchanged with tooth, plaque, and mucosa. Fluoride is loss from saliva by swallowing and splitting (Adapted from Ref. [107]).*

2. FAP formation from supersaturated solutions:

$$10Ca^{2+} + 6PO_4{}^{3-} + 2F^- \rightarrow Ca_{10}(PO_4)_6F_2 \quad (2)$$

3. HAP dissolution and $CaF_2$ formation

$$Ca_{10}(PO_4)_6(OH)_2 + 20F^- \rightarrow 10CaF_2 + 6PO_4{}^{3-} + 2OH^- \quad (3)$$

The first and second reactions occur when the fluoride concentration in the oral fluid is low (typically between 0.01 and 10 ppmF). These reactions lead to the formation of "firmly bound fluoride" as fluoride integrates into the HAP lattice. Fluoride fits snugly into the HAP crystal structure, even better than the hydroxyl group, resulting in lower solubility of the new compound namely FAP compared to HAP. The critical pH (4.5) for densely packed crystals like FAP is slightly lower than the critical pH (5.5) for original HAP. However, in a cariogenic environment, plaque pH levels may drop to 4.5 or lower, and this reduced solubility is insufficient to prevent tooth demineralization [90, 108–111]. Furthermore, studies have demonstrated the occurrence of caries *in vitro* [112] and *in vivo* [113] in shark enameloid, which consists mostly of FAP, even with complete substitution of F for OH in FAP. This supports the notion that a continuous supply of fluoride in oral fluids surrounding tooth enamel during the caries process is more crucial than a high fluoride content in the enamel [114, 115].

The third reaction reveals that in the oral environment with high fluoride concentrations (ranging from 100 to 10,000 ppmF), significant amounts of calcium fluoride ($CaF_2$) or $CaF_2$-like material, rather than FAP, are the predominant products. These high fluoride concentrations are present in topical fluoride treatments, including professional gels and varnishes, fluoride toothpastes, and fluoride mouthwashes [110, 116, 117]. Calcium fluoride formation involves a two-step process. Firstly, calcium ions dissolve from the enamel. Secondly, the dissolved calcium ions bind with applied fluoride, resulting in the formation of calcium fluoride globules [110]. These globules form not only on intact enamel surfaces but also on dental biofilm, acquired salivary pellicle, and demineralized surfaces. The pertinent chemical reactions are depicted in **Figure 35**. In summary, calcium fluoride acts as a pH-controlled fluoride and calcium reservoir that can release free fluoride into the fluids surrounding the tooth, thereby promoting remineralization and hindering demineralization [109, 118].

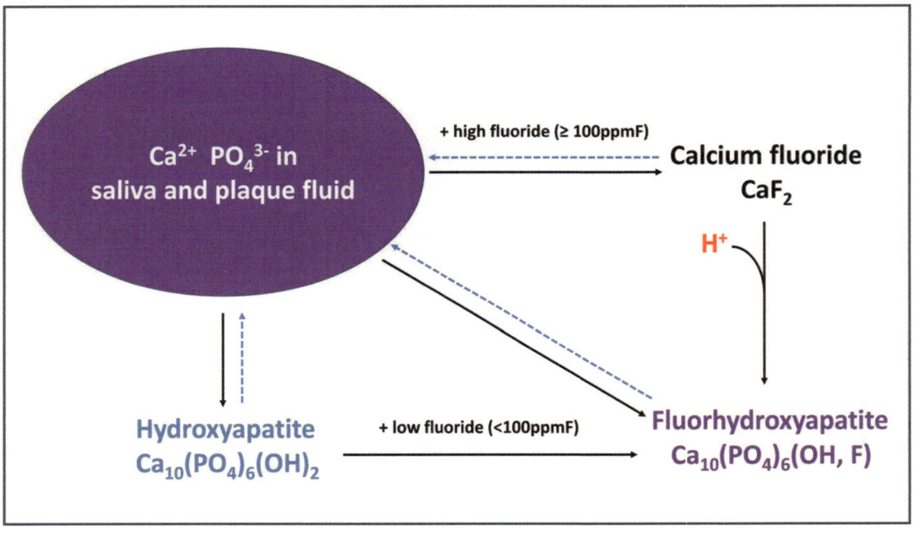


**Figure 35.**
*$CaF_2$ and FAP formation in the oral cavity. FAP was formed during long-term exposure to low fluoride levels (<100 ppmF) in the oral fluid. However, $CaF_2$ is the major or probably the only reaction product on dental hard tissues from short treatments with highly concentrated fluoride (≥ 100 ppmF) agents. Therefore, calcium fluoride acts as a pH-controlled fluoride (and calcium) reservoir (Adapted from Ref. [109]).*

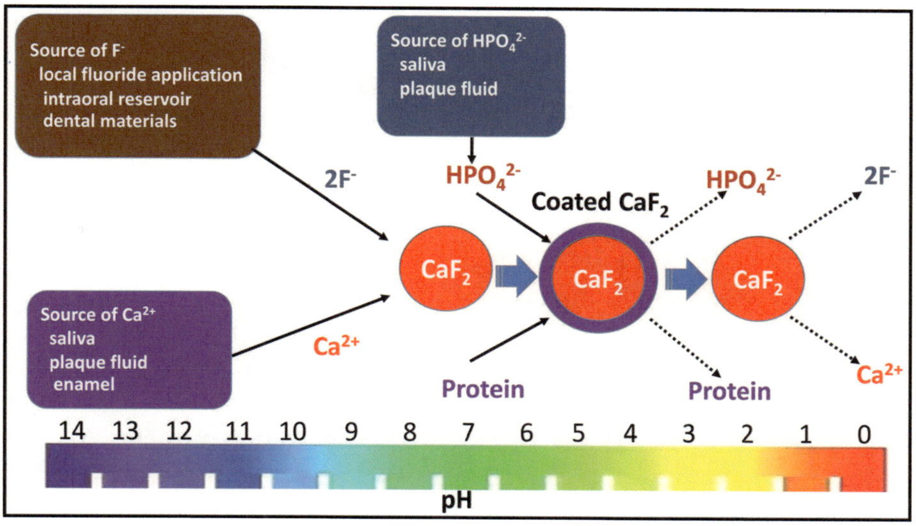


**Figure 36.**
*Formation and decomposition of calcium fluoride-like materials. The calcium fluoride is stabilized by surface adsorption of $HPO_4^{2-}$ and/or also proteins from saliva. This phase can dissolve at pH ≤ 5 and provide fluoride and calcium ions (Adapted from Ref. [90]).*

In summary, while pure $CaF_2$ dissolves readily in water, it does not exist in the oral cavity due to being coated with $HPO_4^{2-}$, proteins, and other saliva-derived substances. This coating enhances the stability of $CaF_2$-like materials by forming a protective film that inhibits solubility. When subjected to acid attacks like those from caries, this protective layer dissolves, releasing calcium and fluoride. Therefore, $CaF_2$-like materials serve as a reservoir for fluoride, releasing it at low pH levels during acid attacks and maintaining stability on tooth surfaces for longer periods at neutral pH levels (**Figure 36**) [90, 119].

## 11.2 Cariostatic mechanisms of fluoride

Currently, it is widely acknowledged that fluorides incorporated into enamel have minimal impact on its solubility. Conversely, small concentrations of fluoride in the vicinity of the tooth exhibit a more potent ability to prevent demineralization compared to fluorides incorporated within the enamel. In such scenarios, fluoride ions partially adsorb to the surface of HAP crystals and maintain a dynamic equilibrium with fluoride ions present in the surrounding fluid. This results in an equilibrium or oversaturation concerning FAP. Adsorbed fluoride ions can attract free calcium ions, primarily sourced from the Stern layer. As a result, these calcium ions bind to available phosphate ions (**Figure 37**), leading to the creation of a remineralized layer akin to FAP on the crystal surface. This veneered surface becomes considerably less soluble than its original state. Importantly, fluoride often facilitates the redeposition of calcium and phosphate ions onto existing crystal remnants rather than the formation of new crystals (**Figure 38**). Additionally, adsorbed fluorides on the HAP crystals are thought to directly shield against demineralization [107, 120]. Due to their significant electronegativity, fluoride ions not only aid in remineralization, as discussed, but can also bind to $H^+$ ions, thereby inhibiting plaque acidity and enamel demineralization [20].

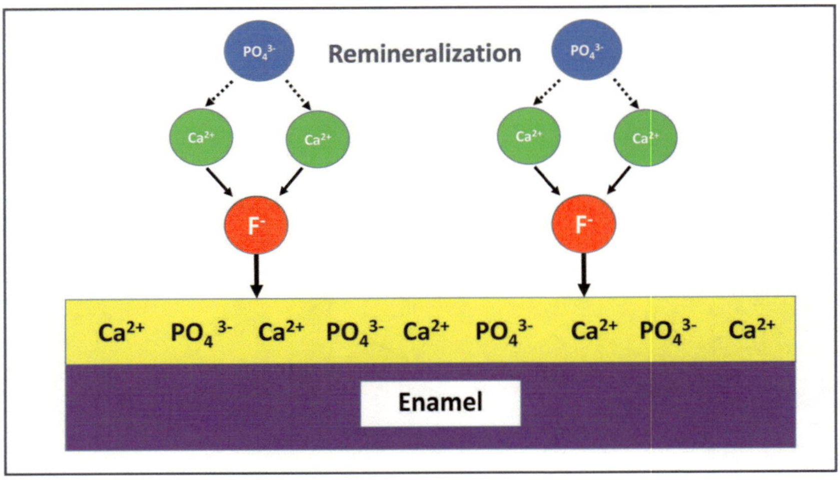


**Figure 37.**
*Enhancement effect of fluoride on calcium phosphate precipitation. Initially, fluoride ions adsorbed to the enamel surface. Then, adsorbed fluoride ions can attract free calcium ions, primarily sourced from the Stern layer. These calcium ions bind to available phosphate ions, leading to the creation of remineralization (Modified from Ref. [120]).*

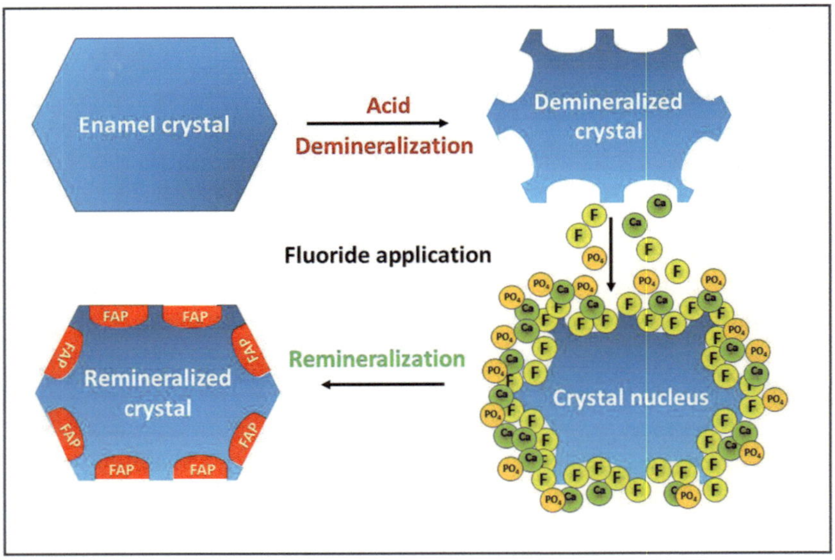


**Figure 38.**
*Schematic representation of demineralization followed by FAP formation. First, fluoride ions adsorbed to the demineralized apatite crystal surface. Consequently, adsorbed fluoride ions attract calcium ions, which attract phosphate ions later, starting to form a FAP-like remineralized veneer on the demineralized crystal surface (Modified from Ref. [107]).*

## 12. Dental erosion

### 12.1 Chemical aspects of erosion

Enamel, which typically withstands exposure to dietary acids, becomes susceptible to dental erosion when subjected to frequent and extended acid exposure. This erosion results from the interaction between tooth surfaces and acids or chelating agents. Primarily, this phenomenon occurs in the absence of plaque [121]. When HAP interacts with erosive solutions, tooth minerals dissolve following the reaction:

$$Ca_{10}(PO_4)_6(OH)_2 + (2 + 3x + 2y + z)\,H^+ \rightarrow 10Ca^{2+} + xH_3PO_4 + yH_2PO_4^{-} + zHPO_4^{2-} + 2H_2O.$$
$$(x + y + z = 6)$$

During erosive challenges, hydrogen ions originating from dietary acids initially target the minerals found in HAP, such as phosphate, hydroxyl, and carbonate ions. This process causes the dissolution of HAP crystallites, releasing calcium ions. Apart from the acid assault resulting from dietary acid exposure, dental erosion can also occur due to the formation of complexes between anions from chelating agents and calcium ions within HAP. For instance, in the citrate ion, two or three COOH groups may have lost their protons, leading to negatively charged sites that attract calcium ions within HAP. Consequently, this results in the dissolution of calcium from the crystal surface [122–124].

The acquired salivary pellicle is a semipermeable membrane [42, 125]. The outer globular layer is the first line of defense against erosive demineralization [126]. Both electron-dense basal and outer globular layers of the pellicle act as a physical barrier to inhibit direct contact between the enamel surface and erosive acids [54, 127]. The semipermeable membrane of an acquired salivary pellicle can delay interaction between erosive acids and the enamel surface [42, 128]. Moreover, the acquired salivary pellicle can modify the transportation of calcium and phosphate ions out and proton ions in at the enamel surface during acid challenge [128, 129]. Therefore, the acid diffusion and enamel dissolution rate are delayed [130]. If the erosive challenge continues, the erosive acids can damage the acquired salivary pellicle and enamel surface [52]. Consequently, proton ions from erosive acids can diffuse through the pellicle membrane [42]. Meanwhile, calcium and phosphate ions at the tooth surface move into the surrounding area [54, 128].

The adsorbed salivary proteins in acquired salivary pellicles, such as PRPs, histatins, carbonic anhydrase, and statherin, have a buffer capacity property [42, 45]. Some salivary proteins have desorbed from the enamel surface to the oral cavity during the erosive challenge for neutralizing erosive acids [131]. Furthermore, these adsorbed salivary proteins, especially statherin, could maintain the level of calcium ions by binding calcium domains of the enamel surface [45, 50]. The acquired salivary pellicle is gradually dissolved after exposure to erosive acids from the outer globular layer to the electron-dense basal layer [42]. Consequently, the thickness of the acquired salivary pellicle is considerably decreased [52]. Therefore, the acquired salivary pellicle acts as physical and chemical protection on the enamel surface against dental erosion [42, 126]. However, the acquired salivary pellicle cannot protect the tooth surface when faced with severe erosive acidity or prolonged exposure time [42].

The acquired salivary pellicle exhibits partial damage after erosive demineralization [56]. The outer globular layer of the acquired salivary pellicle is widely dissolved [52]. Meanwhile, the electron-dense basal layer is partially eroded [52]. The acquired salivary pellicle would be reestablished immediately after erosive demineralization by adsorbed salivary proteins in the oral cavity again [131]. After erosive demineralization, the ultrastructure of acquired salivary pellicle-coated enamel appears noticeably superficially dislodged with localized eroded areas and partially dissolved enamel crystallites [49]. The consequences of enamel erosion are calcium and phosphate loss, surface roughness, and surface microhardness loss in enamel [132]. The preventive effect of the

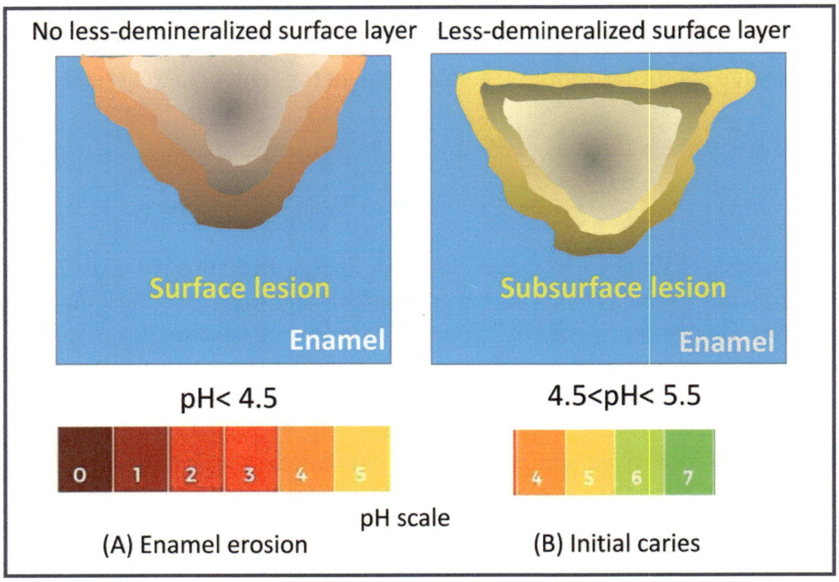


**Figure 39.**
*Schematic illustration of the difference between caries and erosion lesions. At pH levels between 4.5 and 5.5, HAP tends to dissolve, whereas FAP will be formed. Thus, the subsurface lesion is observed in the initial carious lesion. In contrast, surface-softened lesions (erosion) occur when the pH level is lower than 4.5 due to the dissolution of both HAP and FAP (Adapted from Ref. [134]).*

acquired salivary pellicle depends on the maturation stage, the thickness and compositions of the acquired salivary pellicle, the concentration of erosive acids, and the exposure time of erosive acids [43, 130, 131, 133].

### 12.2 Histological features of erosive enamel

Between pH levels of 4.5–5.5, HAP is prone to dissolution, potentially leading to the formation of FAP and the initiation of early carious lesions. Conversely, when the pH drops below the critical value for FAP (pH $\leq$ 4.5), both HAP and FAP may dissolve, resulting in dental erosion. Unlike the process of initial caries, where demineralization creates a subsurface lesion with a relatively intact surface initially, dental erosion predominantly impacts the surface layer (**Figure 39**) [86, 121, 134, 135]. Ultrastructure of the naturally eroded enamel showed small, shallow, irregular depressions with a characteristic honeycomb-like or pitted appearance (**Figure 40A**). At higher magnification, small globules occurring singly or as aggregates were seen in erosive areas (**Figure 40B**) [136]. These appearances were also found in the experimental erosive enamel. After 7–15 days of immersion in the cola-type soft drink (pH 2.35), there was an accentuated demineralization of the entire enamel surface, being more pronounced on the interprismatic portion [137].

## 13. Concluding remarks

Enamel's structural integrity relies on a meticulously organized hierarchical arrangement, spanning various dimensions, from the atomic level with HAP, to nanoscale crystallites, to microscale enamel rods, and ultimately to the tooth's entire

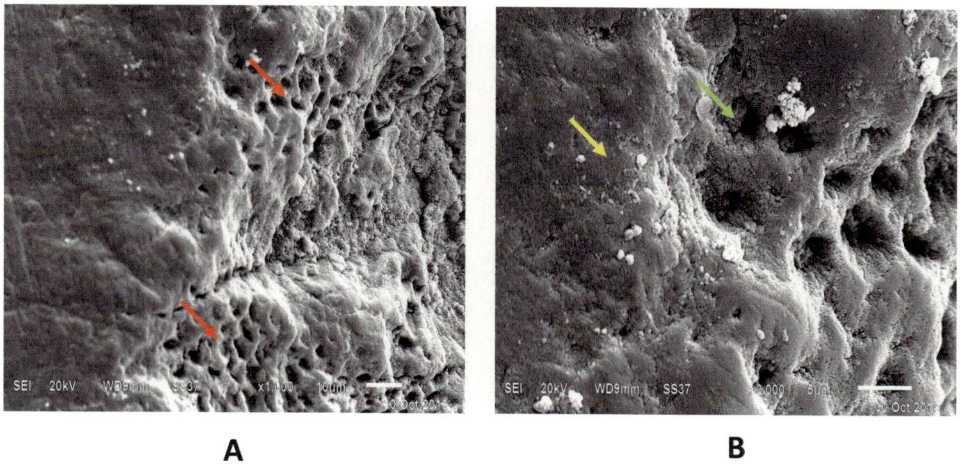


**Figure 40.**
*SEM of naturally eroded enamel at the initial stage. (A) The eroded area shows a rough and irregular surface in association with a honeycomb-like surface (red arrow) (original magnification x 1000; bar = 10 μm). (B) At higher magnification, the eroded enamel shows loosely packed globular crystals (green arrow), whereas the adjacent normal-appearing enamel surface consists of densely packed globular crystals (yellow arrow). Original magnification x 5000; bar = 5 μm.*

surface. While HAP is composed of 10 calcium ions, 6 phosphate ions, and 2 hydroxyl ions $[Ca_{10}(PO_4)_6(OH)_2]$, enamel deviates from stoichiometric HAP due to deficiencies in primary constituents such as $Ca^{2+}$, $PO_4^{3-}$, and $OH^-$, and the inclusion of ions such as $CO_3^{2-}$, $HPO_4^{2-}$, and trace elements. Under normal conditions, the tooth surface is exposed to saliva, oral bacteria, fluoride from oral products, and dietary acids. Upon contact with saliva, tooth surfaces adsorb salivary proteins, forming an acquired salivary pellicle. The oral cavity hosts diverse oral microorganisms, forming biofilms on dental and mucosal surfaces. Salivary components within the acquired salivary pellicle play a pivotal role in initial bacterial adherence. While dental biofilms contribute to host well-being, disruptions in this relationship can lead to oral diseases such as dental caries and periodontal diseases. According to the Ecological Plaque Hypothesis, dental caries result from microbiota imbalance due to ecological stress, leading to an abundance of cariogenic bacteria. In cariogenic conditions, reduced concentrations of $OH^-$ and $PO_4^{3-}$ in plaque fluids, and potentially saliva, cause the Ip in plaque fluids to fall below the Ksp of HAP, initiating enamel dissolution. However, it is crucial to recognize that the caries process involves cycles of demineralization and remineralization. Initial carious lesions manifest as subsurface lesions with a clinical appearance resembling white spot lesions. SEM of initial caries exhibits accentuation of the perikymata, deep focal holes, and broadening of interprismatic spaces. Mineral dissolution was markedly observed at prism cores, compared to prism borders.

Currently, it is widely acknowledged that $CaF_2$ is vital in caries prevention. Formation occurs when fluoride concentration around enamel surpasses 100 ppmF. However, the ability to form calcium fluoride-like materials during brief intraoral exposure is limited, and these compounds are swiftly lost after using fluoride-containing oral products. The tooth surface may be exposed to acidic diets, with prolonged exposure leading to dental erosion. Erosion involves the chemical loss of dental hard tissue, unrelated to bacterial action, induced by hydrogen ions and/or chelating agents. It typically occurs when fluid pH around the tooth surface drops below 4.5, causing FAP and HAP dissolution under acidic conditions. Additionally, several proteins in saliva and the acquired salivary pellicle may offer protection against dental erosion.

## Acknowledgements

The authors would like to thank Christian Estacio, International College of Dentistry, Walailak University, for critically reading the text.

## Author details

Sittichai Koontongkaew[1*], Kusumawadee Utispan[2],
Darren Dhananthat Chawhuaveang[2,3], Ollie Yiru Yu[3] and Rattapong Worawongvasu[1]

1 International College of Dentistry, Walailak University, Bangkok, Thailand

2 Faculty of Dentistry, Thammasat University, Pathum Thani, Thailand

3 Faculty of Dentistry, The University of Hong Kong, Hong Kong, SAR, China

*Address all correspondence to: koontongkaew@gmail.com

## References

[1] Klimuszko E, Orywal K, Sierpinska T, Sidun J, Golebiewska M. Evaluation of calcium and magnesium contents in tooth enamel without any pathological changes: *In vitro* preliminary study. Odontology. 2018;**106**:369-376

[2] LeGeros. Calcium-phosphates in enamel dentin and bone. Monographs in Oral Science. 1991;**15**:108-129

[3] Gil-Bona A, Bidlack FB. Tooth enamel and its dynamic protein matrix. International Journal of Molecular Sciences. 2020;**21**:4458

[4] Shahmoradi M, Bertassoni LE, Elfallah HM, Swain M. Fundamental structure and properties of enamel, dentin and cementum. In: Ben-Nissan B, editor. Advances in Calcium Phosphate Biomaterials. Berlin: Spinger; 2014. pp. 511-547

[5] Nikiforuk G. The nature of tooth substance. In: Nikiforuk G, editor. Understanding Dental Carie: Etiology and Mechanisms, Basic and Clinical Aspects. Basel: Karger; 1985. pp. 83-118

[6] Berkovitz BKB, Holland GR, Moxham BJ. Enamel. In: Berkovitz BKB, Holland GR, Moxham BJ, editors. Oral Anatomy, Histology and Embryology. London: Elsevier; 2018. pp. 123-143

[7] de Siqueira MT, Palma-Dibb RG, de Oliveira HF, Garcia Paula-Silva FW, Nelson-Filho P, da Silva RA, et al. The effect of radiation therapy on the mechanical and morphological properties of the enamel and dentin of deciduous teeth–An in vitro study. Radiation Oncology. 2014;**9**:30

[8] Pandya M, Diekwisch TGH. Enamel biomimetics-fiction or future of dentistry. International Journal of Oral Science. 2019;**11**:8

[9] Nanci A. Enamel: Composition, formation, and structure. In: Nanci A, editor. Ten Cate's Oral-Histology: Development, Structure, and Function. 7th ed. St. Louis: Elsevier; 2008. pp. 141-190

[10] Chiego DJ. Enamel. In: Chiego DJ, editor. Essentials of Oral Histology and Embryology: A Clinical Approach. 5th ed. St. Louis, Missouri: Elsevier; 2019. pp. 88-96

[11] White SN, Luo W, Paine ML, Fong H, Sarikaya M, Snead ML. Biological organization of hydroxyapatite crystallites into a fibrous continuum toughens and control anisotropy in human enamel. Journal of Dental Research. 2001;**80**: 321-326

[12] Desai D. Enamel. In: Kumar GS, editor. Orban's Oral Histology and Embryology. New Delhi: Elsevier; 2015. pp. 40-73

[13] Pandya M, Lin T, Li L, Allen MJ, Jin T, Luan X, et al. Posttranslational amelogenin processing and changes in matrix assembly during enamel development. Frontiers in Physiology. 2017;**8**:790

[14] Habelitz S. Materials engineering by ameloblasts. Journal of Dental Research. 2015;**94**:759-767

[15] Xia J, Tian ZR, Hua L, Chen L, Zhou Z, Qian L, et al. Enamel crystallite strength and wear: Nanoscale responses of teeth to chewing loads. Journal of the Royal Society, Interface. 2017;**14**: 20170456

[16] Horiuchi N, Endo J, Nozaki K, Nakamura M, Nagai A, Katayama K, et al. Dielectric evaluation of fluorine substituted hydroxyapatite. Journal of the Ceramic Society of Japan. 2013;**121**: 770-774

[17] Li L, Pan H, Tao J, Xu X, Mao C, Gu X, et al. Repair of enamel by using hydroxyapatite nanoparticles as the building blocks. Journal of Materials Chemistry. 2008;**18**:4079-4084

[18] Combes C, Cazalbou S, Rey C. Apatite biominerals. Minerals. 2016;**6**:34

[19] Simmer JP, Hardy NC, Chinoy AF, Bartlett JD, Hu JC. How fluoride protects dental enamel from demineralization. Journal of International Society of Preventive & Community Dentistry. 2020;**10**:134-141

[20] Zimmer S, Jahn KR, Barrthel CR. Recommendations for the use of fluoride in caries prevention. Oral Health & Preventive Dentistry. 2003;**1**:45-51

[21] Tchijo T, Yamachita Y, Terashima T. Observation on structure features and characteristics of biological apatite crystals 5. Three-dimensional on ultrastructure of human enamel crystals. The Bulletin of Tokyo Medical and Dental University. 1993;**40**: 135-146

[22] Rivera-Munoz EM. Hydroxyapatite-based materials: Synthesis and characterization. In: Fazel-Rezal E, editor. Biomedical Engineering - Frontiers and Challenges. London: InTechOpen; 2011. pp. 75-98

[23] Verbeeck RMH. Minerals in human enamel and dentin. In: Driessens FCM, Wolgens JHM, editors. Tooth Development and Caries. Boca Raton, Florida: CRC Press; 1986. pp. 95-152

[24] Young RA. Biological apatite vs hydroxyapatite at the atomic level. Clinical Orthopaedics and Related Research. 1975;**113**:249-262

[25] Oliveira M, Mansur HS. Synthetic tooth enamel: SEM characterization of a fluoride hydroxyapatite coating for dentistry application. Materials Research. 2007;**10**:115-118

[26] Solhy A, Amer W, Karkouri M, Tahir R, El Bouari A, Fihri A, et al. Bi-functional modified-phosphate catalyzed the synthesis of α-α′-(EE)-bis (benzylidene)-cycloalkanones: Microwave versus conventional-heating. Journal of Molecular Catalysis A: Chemical. 2011;**336**:8-15

[27] Paterlini V, Bettinelli M, Rizzi R, El Khouri A, Rossi M, Della Ventura G, et al. Characterization and luminescence of $Eu^{3+}$- and $Gd^{3+}$-doped hydroxyapatite $Ca_{10}(PO_4)_6(OH)_2$. Crystals. 2020;**10**:806

[28] Chappard D, Bizot P, Mabilleau G, Hubert L. Aluminum and bone: Review of new clinical circumstances associated with $Al^{3+}$ deposition in the calcified matrix of bone. Morphologie. 2016;**100**: 95-105

[29] Malcangi G, Patano A, Morolla R, De Santis M, Piras F, Settanni V, et al. Analysis of dental enamel remineralization: A systematic review of technique comparisons. Bioengineering (Basel). 2023;**10**:472

[30] Elliott JC. Structure, crystal chemistry and density of enamel apatites. Ciba Foundation Symposium. 1997;**205**:54-67

[31] Clasen ABS, Ruyter LE. Quantitative determination of type A and type B carbonate in human deciduous and permanent enamel by mean of Fourrier transform infrared spectrometry.

Advances in Dental Research. 1997;**11**: 523-527

[32] Jin X, Yang W, Gao X, Li Z. Analysis and modeling of the complex dielectric constant of bound water with application in soil microwave remote sensing. Remote Sensing. 2020;**12**:3544

[33] Arends J, Jongebloed WL. The enamel substrate-characteristics of the enamel surface. Swedish Dental Journal. 1977;**1**:215-224

[34] Orij R, Brul S, Smits GJ. Intracellular pH is a tightly controlled signal in yeast. Biochimica et Biophysica Acta. 2011; **1810**:933-944

[35] Arends J, Nelson DGA, Dijkman AG, Jongebloed WL. Effects of various fluorides on enamel structure and chemistry. In: Guggenheim B, editor. Cariology Today. Basel: Karger; 1984. pp. 245-258

[36] de Almeida PDV, Grégio AMT, Machado MAN, et al. Saliva composition and functions: A comprehensive review. The Journal of Contemporary Dental Practice. 2008;**9**:072-080

[37] Hick J, Garcia-Godoy F, Flaitz C. Biological factors in dental caries: Role of saliva and dental plaque in the dynamic process of demineralization and remineralization (part 1). The Journal of Clinical Pediatric Dentistry. 2003;**28**: 47-52

[38] Lamont RJ, Koo H, Hajishengallis G. The oral microbiota: Dynamic communities and host interactions. Nature Reviews. Microbiology. 2018;**16**: 745-759

[39] Marsh PD. Dental plaque as a biofilm and a microbial community - Implications for health and disease. BMC Oral Health. 2006;**6**:S14

[40] Naumova EA, Kuehnl P, Hertenstein P, Markovic L, Jordan RA, Gaengler P, et al. Fluoride bioavailability in saliva and plaque. BMC Oral Health. 2012;**12**:3

[41] Lussi A, Jaeggi T, Zero D. The role of diet in the aetiology of dental erosion. Caries Research. 2004;**38**(Suppl. 1): 34-44

[42] Hannig M, Hannig C. The pellicle and erosion. Monographs in Oral Science. 2014;**25**:206-214

[43] Chawhuaveang DD, Yu OY, Yin IX, Lam WY, Mei ML, Chu CH. Acquired salivary pellicle and oral diseases: A literature review. Journal of Dental Sciences. 2021;**16**:523-529

[44] Sieber KR, Schmidt C, Baumann T, Lussi A, Carvalho TS. Acquired enamel pellicle modification with casein and mucin in different concentrations and its impact on initial dental erosion. Caries Research. 2019;**53**:457-466

[45] Mutahar M, O'Toole S, Carpenter G, Bartlett D, Andiappan M, Moazzez R. Reduced statherin in acquired enamel pellicle on eroded teeth compared to healthy teeth in the same subjects: An in-vivo study. PLoS One. 2017;**12**:e0183660

[46] Finke M, Parker DM, Jandt KD. Influence of soft drinks on the thickness and morphology of *in situ* acquired pellicle layer on enamel. Journal of Colloid and Interface Science. 2002;**251**: 263-270

[47] Siqueira WL, Custodio W, McDonald EE. New insights into the composition and functions of the acquired enamel pellicle. Journal of Dental Research. 2012;**91**:1110-1118

[48] Kensche A, Reich M, Hannig C, Kummerer K, Hannig M. Modification of

the lipid profile of the initial oral biofilm in situ using linseed oil as mouthwash. Nutrients. 2021;**13**:989

[49] Hannig M, Fiebiger M, Güntzer M, Döbert A, Zimehl R, Nekrashevych Y. Protective effect of the in situ formed short-term salivary pellicle. Archives of Oral Biology. 2004;**49**:903-910

[50] Baumann T, Bereiter R, Lussi A, Carvalho T. The effect of different salivary calcium concentrations on the erosion protection conferred by the salivary pellicle. Scientific Reports. 2017; **7**:12999

[51] Nekrashevych Y, Stösser L. Protective influence of experimentally formed salivary pellicle on enamel erosion. Caries Research. 2003;**37**: 225-231

[52] Hannig C, Berndt D, Hoth-Hannig W, Hannig M. The effect of acidic beverages on the ultrastructure of the acquired pellicle—An *in situ* study. Archives of Oral Biology. 2009;**54**: 518-526

[53] Delecrode T, Siqueira W, Zaidan F, Bellini M, Moffa E, Mussi M, et al. Identification of acid-resistant proteins in acquired enamel pellicle. Journal of Dentistry. 2015;**43**:1470-1475

[54] Vukosavljevic D, Custodio W, Buzalaf RMA, et al. Acquired pellicle as a modulator for dental erosion. Archives of Oral Biology. 2014;**59**:631-638

[55] Cheaib Z, Lussi A. Impact of acquired enamel pellicle modification on initial dental erosion. Caries Research. 2011;**45**:107-112

[56] Lussi A, Bossen A, Höschele C, Beyeler B, Megert B, Meier C, et al. Effects of enamel abrasion, salivary pellicle, and measurement angle on the optical assessment of dental erosion. Journal of Biomedical Optics. 2012;**17**: 097009

[57] Gibbon RJ, van Houte J. Bacterial adherence and the formation of dental plaque. In: Beachey EH, editor. Bacterial Adherence. London: Chapman and Hall; 1980. pp. 61-104

[58] Lebeaux D, Ghigo JM, Beloin C. Biofilm-related infection: bridging the gap between clinical management and fundamental aspects of recalcitrance toward antibiotics. Microbiology and Molecular Biology Reviews. 2014;**78**: 510-543

[59] Marsh PD, Bradshaw DJ. Dental plaque as a biofilm. Journal of Industrial Microbiology. 1995;**15**:169-175

[60] Singh S, Singh SK, Chowdhury I, Singh R. Understanding the mechanism of bacterial biofilms resistance to antimicrobial agents. The Open Microbiology Journal. 2017;**11**:53-62

[61] Bowen WH, Koo H. Biology of *Streptococcus mutans*-derived glucosyltransferases: Role in extracellular matrix formation of cariogenic biofilms. Caries Research. 2011;**45**:69-86

[62] Rickard AH, Gilbert P, High NJ, Kolenbrander PE, Handley PS. Bacterial coaggregation: An integral process in the development of multi-species biofilms. Trends in Microbiology. 2003;**11**:94-100

[63] Jakubovics NS, Yassin SA, Rickard AH. Community interactions of oral streptococci. Advances in Applied Microbiology. 2014;**87**:43-110

[64] Hannig C, Hannig M. The oral cavity–A key system to understand substratum-dependent bioadhesion on

solid surfaces in man. Clinical Oral Investigations. 2009;**13**:123-139

[65] Huang R, Li M, Gregory RL. Bacterial interactions in dental biofilm. Virulence. 2011;**2**:435-444

[66] Marsh PD. Dental biofilm in health and disease. In: Goldberg M, editor. Understanding Dental Caries: From Pathogenesis to Prevention and Therapy. Switzerland: Springer; 2016. pp. 41-52

[67] Ribeiro M, Simões M. Oral biofilms. In: Simoes M, Borges A, Simoes LC, editors. Recent Trends in Biofilm Science and Technology. London: Elsevier; 2020. pp. 89-99

[68] Kolenbrander PE, Palmer RJ Jr, Periasamy S, Jakubovics NS. Oral multispecies biofilm development and the key role of cell-cell distance. Nature Reviews. Microbiology. 2010;**8**:471-480

[69] Mahajan A, Singh B, Kashyap D, Kumar A, Mahajan P. Interspecies communication and periodontal disease. Scientific World Journal. 2013;**2013**: 765434

[70] Relucenti M, Familiari G, Donfrancesco O, Taurino M, Li X, Chen R, et al. Microscopy methods for biofilm imaging: Focus on SEM and VP-SEM pros and cons. Biology. 2021;**10**:51

[71] Diaz PI, Valm AM. Microbial interactions in oral communities mediate emergent biofilm properties. Journal of Dental Research. 2020;**99**:18-25

[72] Karpinski TM, Szkaradkiewicz AK. Chlorhexidine–pharmaco-biological activity and application. European Review for Medical and Pharmacological Sciences. 2015;**19**:1321-1326

[73] Newbrun E. Substrate: diet and caries. In: Newbrun E, editor. Cariology. 3rd ed. Chicago: Quintessence; 1989. pp. 99-134

[74] Nishimura J, Saito T, Yoneyama H, Lan Bai L, Okumura K, Isogai E. Biofilm formation by *Streptococcus mutans* and related bacteria. Advances in Applied Microbiology. 2012;**2**:208-215

[75] Paes Leme AF, Koo H, Bellato CM, Bedi G, Cury JA. The role of sucrose in cariogenic dental biofilm formation–New insight. Journal of Dental Research. 2006;**85**:878-887

[76] Ho MH, Lamont RJ, Xie H. A novel peptidic inhibitor derived from *Streptococcus cristatus* ArcA attenuates virulence potential of *Porphyromonas gingivalis*. Scientific Reports. 2017;7: 16217

[77] Wu J, Xie H. Role of arginine deiminase of *Streptococcus cristatus* in *Porphyromonas gingivalis* colonization. Antimicrobial Agents and Chemotherapy. 2010;**54**:4694-4698

[78] Zhu L, Kreth J. The role of hydrogen peroxide in environmental adaptation of oral microbial communities. Oxidative Medicine and Cellular Longevity. 2012; **2012**:717843

[79] Marsh PD. Are dental diseases examples of ecological catastrophes? Microbiology (Reading). 2003;**149**: 279-294

[80] Selwitz RH, Ismail AI, Pitts NB. Dental caries. Lancet. 2007; **369**:51-59

[81] Rosier BT, De Jager M, Zaura E, Krom BP. Historical and contemporary hypotheses on the development of oral diseases: Are we there yet? Frontiers in Cellular and Infection Microbiology. 2014;**4**:92

[82] Sanchez MC, Velapatino A, Llama-Palacios A, Valdes A, Cifuentes A, Ciudad MJ, et al. Metataxonomic and metabolomic evidence of biofilm homeostasis disruption related to caries: An in vitro study. Molecular Oral Microbiology. 2022;**37**:81-96

[83] Thanetchaloempong W, Koontongkaew S, Utispan K. Fixed orthodontic treatment increases cariogenicity and virulence gene expression in dental biofilm. Journal of Clinical Medicine. 2022;**11**:5860

[84] Anderson P, Creanor S. Enamel. In: Creanor S, editor. Essential clinical oral biology. Iowa: John Wiley & Son; 2016. pp. 24-33

[85] Zero DT. Dental caries process. Dental Clinics of North America. 1999; **43**:635-664

[86] Fejerskove O, Larsen MJ. Demineralization and remineralization: The key to understanding clinical manifestations of dental caries. In: Fejerskove O, Nyvad B, Kidd E, editors. Dental Caries: The Disease and Its Clinical Management. 3rd ed. Oxford: Wiley Blackwell; 2015. pp. 155-170

[87] Dawes C. What is the critical pH and why does a tooth dissolve in acid? Journal of the Canadian Dental Association. 2003;**69**:722-724

[88] Verdier JM, Dussol B, Berland Y, et al. Protein inhibitors of calcium salt crystal growth in saliva, bile and pancreatic juice. Scanning Microscopy. 1993;**7**:1017-1030

[89] Schlesinger DH, Hay D, Levine MJ. Complete primary structure of statherin, a potent inhibitor of calcium phosphate precipitation, from the saliva of the monkey, *Macaca arctoides*. International Journal of Peptide and Protein Research. 1989;**34**:374-380

[90] Lussi A, Hellwig E, Klimek J. Fluoride-mode of action and recommendations for use. Schweizer Monatsschrift für Zahnmedizin. 2012; **112**:1030-1036

[91] Chow LC. Diffusion of ions between two solutions saturated with respect to hydroxyapatie: A possible mechanism for subsurface demineralization of teeth. Journal of Research of the National Institute of Standards and Technology. 2010;**115**:217-224

[92] Carey CM. Remineralization of early enamel lesions with apatite-forming salt. Dentistry Journal (Basel). 2023;**11**:182

[93] Aoba T. Solubility properties of human tooth mineral and pathogenesis of dental caries. Oral Diseases. 2004;**10**: 249-257

[94] Hicks J, Garcia-Godoy F, Flaitz C. Biological factors in dental caries enamel structure and the caries process in the dynamic process of demineralization and remineralization (part 2). The Journal of Clinical Pediatric Dentistry. 2004;**28**: 119-124

[95] Aiswarya A, Wael II, Abdullah AM, Reghunathan P, Sukumaran A. Demineralization and remineralization dynamics and dental caries. In: Rusu L-C, Ardelean LC, editors. Dental Caries-The Selection of Restoration Methods and Restorative Materials. Rijeka: IntechOpen; 2022

[96] Warreth A. Dental caries and its management. International Journal of Dentistry. 2023;**2023**:9365845

[97] Siddiqui S, Anderson P, Al-Jawad M. Recovery of crystallographic texture in

remineralized dental enamel. PLoS One. 2014;**9**:e108879

[98] Nikiforuk G. The caries process — Morphological and chemical events. In: Nikiforuk G, editor. Understanding Dental Caries: Etiology and Mechanisms, Basic and Clinical Aspects. Basel: S. Karger; 1985. pp. 261-289

[99] Silverstone LM, Hick MJ, Featherstone MJ. Dynamic factors affecting initiation and progression in human dental enamel, part I. The dynamic nature of enamel caries. Quintessence International. 1988;**19**:683-711

[100] Goldberg M. The early enamel carious lesion. In: Goldberg M, editor. Understanding Dental Caries: From Pathogenesis to Prevention and Therapy. Switzerland: Springer; 2016. pp. 29-39

[101] Flemming J, Hannig C, Hannig M. Caries management-the role of surface interactions in de- and remineralization-processes. Journal of Clinical Medicine. 2022;**11**

[102] Arends J, Christoffersen J. The nature of early caries lesions in enamel. Journal of Dental Research. 1986;**65**:2-11

[103] Melrose CA, Appleton J, Lovius BB. A scanning electron microscopic study of early enamel caries formed in vivo beneath orthodontic bands. British Journal of Orthodontics. 1996; **23**:43-47

[104] Worawongvasu R. A scanning electron microscopic study of enamel surfaces of incipient caries. Ultrastructural Pathology. 2015;**39**:408-412

[105] Brading MG, Marsh PD. The oral environment: The challenge for antimicrobials in oral care products. International Dental Journal. 2003;**53**: 353-362

[106] Ekstrand KJ, Oliveby A. Fluoride in the oral environment. Acta Odontologica Scandinavica. 1999;**57**:330-333

[107] ten Cate JM. Contemporary perspective on the use of fluoride products in caries prevention. British Dental Journal. 2013;**214**:161-167

[108] Rosin-Grget K, Peros K, Sutej I, Basic K. The cariostatic mechanisms of fluoride. Acta Medica Academica. 2013; **42**:179-188

[109] ten Cate JM. Current concepts on the theories of the mechanism of action of fluoride. Acta Odontologica Scandinavica. 1999;**57**:325-329

[110] Buzalaf MAR, Pessan JP, Honorio HM, et al. Mechanism of action of fluoride for caries control. Monographs in Oral Science. 2011;**22**:97-114

[111] ten Cate JM, Buzalaf MAR. Fluoride mode of action: Once there was an observant dentist. Journal of Dental Research. 2019;**98**:725-730

[112] LeGeros RZ, Silverstone LM, Daculsi G, et al. *In vitro* caries like lesion formation in F-containing tooth enamel. Journal of Dental Research. 1983;**62**:138

[113] Ogaard B, Rolla C, Ruben J, et al. Microradiographic study of demineraiization of shark enamel in a human caries model. Scandinavian Journal of Dental Research. 1988;**96**: 209-211

[114] Larsen MJ, von der Fehr FR, Birkeland JM. Effect of fluoride on the saturation of an acetate buffer with respect to hydroxyapatite. Archives of Oral Biology. 1976;**21**:723-728

[115] ten Cate JM, Featherstone JDB. Mechanistic aspects of the interactions

between fluoride and dental enamel. Critical Reviews in Oral Biology and Medicine. 1991;**2**:283-296

[116] Navarro M, Monte Aito LA, Cruz RA, et al. Calcium fluoride uptake by human enamel after use of fluoridated mouth rinse. Brazilian Dental Journal. 2001;**12**:178-182

[117] Ogaard B. $CaF_2$ formation: Cariostatic properties and factors of enhancing the effects. Caries Research. 2001;**35**:40-44

[118] Rosin-Grget K, Lineir I. Current concept on the anticaries fluoride mechanism of the action. Collegium Antropologicum. 2001;**25**:703-712

[119] Rolla G. On the role of calcium fluoride in the cariostatic mechanism of fluoride. Acta Odontologica Scandinavica. 1988;**46**:341-345

[120] Featherstone JDB. Dental caries: A dynamic disease process. Australian Dental Journal. 2008;**53**:286-291

[121] Lussi A, Schlueter N, Rakhmatullina E, Ganss C. Dental erosion-An overview with emphasis on chemical and histopathological aspects. Caries Research. 2011;**45**(Suppl. 1):2-12

[122] Featherstone JDB, Lussi A. Understanding the chemistry of dental erosion. Monographs in Oral Science. 2006;**20**:66-76

[123] Shellis RP, Featherstone JDB, Lussi A. Understanding the chemistry of dental erosion. Monographs in Oral Science. 2014;**25**:163-179

[124] Goldberg M. Enamel softening (dental erosion). In: Goldberg M, editor. Understanding Dental Caries: From Pathogenesis to Prevention and Therapy. Switzerland: Springer; 2016. pp. 11-17

[125] Hara AT, Ando M, González-Cabezas C, Cury JA, Serra MC, Zero DT. Protective effect of the dental pellicle against erosive challenges *in situ*. Journal of Dental Research. 2006;**85**:612-616

[126] Wetton S, Hughes J, West N, Addy M. Exposure time of enamel and dentine to saliva for protection against erosion: A study *in vitro*. Caries Research. 2006;**40**: 213-217

[127] Hara AT, Zero DT. The potential of saliva in protecting against dental erosion. Monographs in Oral Science. 2014;**25**:197-205

[128] Bartlett D, German M, Moazzez R. The presence of acquired enamel pellicle changes acid-induced erosion from dissolution to a softening process. Scientific Reports. 2017;**7**:10920

[129] Hannig C, Becker K, Häusler N, Hoth-Hannig W, Attin T, Hannig M. Protective effect of the in situ pellicle on dentin erosion–An ex vivo pilot study. Archives of Oral Biology. 2007;**52**: 444-449

[130] Moazzez RV, Austin RS, Rojas-Serrano M, Carpenter G, Cotroneo E, Proctor G, et al. Comparison of the possible protective effect of the salivary pellicle of individuals with and without erosion. Caries Research. 2014;**48**:57-62

[131] Jensdottir T, Holbrook P, Nauntofte B, Buchwald C, Bardow A. Immediate erosive potential of cola drinks and orange juices. Journal of Dental Research. 2006;**85**:226-230

[132] Hove HL, Holme B, Young A, et al. The erosion-inhibiting effect of $TiF_4$, $SnF_2$, and NaF solutions on pellicle-covered enamel *in vitro*. Acta Odontologica Scandinavica. 2007;**65**: 259-264

[133] Stroici C, Daraba O, Cojocariu A, Bîrgaoanu A, Sachelarie L, Nazarie S. Protective role of acquired pellicle on enamel erosion. International Journal of Medical Dentistry. 2012;**2**:272-275

[134] Buzalaf MA, Hannas AR, Magalhaes AC, Rios D, Honorio HM, Delbem AC. pH-cycling models for *in vitro* evaluation of the efficacy of fluoridated dentifrices for caries control: Strengths and limitations. Journal of Applied Oral Science. 2010;**18**:316-334

[135] Larsen MJ. On the chemical and physical nature of erosions and caries lesions in dental enamel. Caries Research. 1991;**25**:323-329

[136] Worawongvasu R. Scanning electron microscope characterization of erosive enamel in human teeth. Ultrastructural Pathology. 2015;**39**: 395-401

[137] Torres CP, Chinelatti MA, Gomes-Silva JM, et al. Surface and subsurface erosion of primary enamel by acid beverage over time. Brazilian Dental Journal. 2010;**21**:337-345

Chapter 3

# Hereditary Tooth Anomalies: Amelogenesis Imperfecta, Dentinogenesis Imperfecta, Dentine Dysplasia

*Abubaker El Elhaj*


## Abstract

Amelogenesis imperfecta (AI), dentinogenesis imperfecta (DI), and dentin dysplasia (DD) are hereditary illnesses that affect the growth and architecture of teeth's hard tissues (enamel and dentine). These diseases present clinical symptoms such as tooth discoloration, enamel/dentine abnormalities, and enhanced tooth sensitivity. AI is defined by teeth enamel flaws, while DI is characterized by anomalies in dentin development, leading to opalescent or yellow-brown teeth, greater translucency, and a higher risk of fractures. DD is less prevalent than AI or DI. The genetic basis of DD, DI, and AI is derived from gene alterations. Mutations in the DSPP, DMP1, COL1A1, and COL1A2 genes are linked to DI, while the DSPP, DMP1, and COL1A2 genes are the cause of DD. Family genetic history was used to detect genetic mutation and confirm diagnosis, with treatment options including endodontic therapy, restorative dentistry, and preventative treatments as in fluoride therapy and oral hygiene guidelines. Early diagnosis and effective treatment are essential for enhancing oral health and quality of life.


**Keywords:** amelogenesis imperfecta, dentinogenesis imperfecta, dentine dysplasia, gene mutation, tooth sensitivity

## 1. Introduction

Tooth development anomalies, particularly those related to the enamel and dentin complex, can negatively impact oral health. Genetic and modern lifestyle factors influence enamel and dentin development, such as acidic foods, stress, and inadequate dental care. Hereditary and environmental influences interact to dental abnormalities, leading to Amelogenesis Imperfecta (AI), Dentinogenesis Imperfecta (DI) and odontodysplasia, these conditions could result in tooth sensitivity, structural flaws in the teeth, or complete loss, which would impair mastication and the facial esthetics. Congenital anomalies in enamel and dentin in permanent and deciduous teeth can cause symptoms alone or in systemic syndromes, posing challenges to basic science research and clinical care [1]. Dental agenesis is the most prevalent developmental anomaly in humans and is often linked to multiple other oral abnormalities as in growth hormone-deficient children have tooth anomalies that affect tooth size and enamel growth [2]. Similarly, systemic illnesses such as ectodermal dysplasia are linked to hypodontia or oligodontia and may have etiological involvement from both genetic and environmental sources . The abnormalities known as dental anomalies are associated with genetic mutations in dentin and enamel structure, such as the altered dentin sialophosphoprotein (DSPP) gene [3]. In this context, there is prominent cervical constriction, bulbous crowns, pulpal obliteration, and a crescent-shaped remnant of amelogenesis imperfecta in major teeth, which also include pulp stones, dentin dysplasia type II. Dental agenesis is divided into acquired and developmental anomalies, causing various disorders [4]. Developmental anomalies, characterized by variations in tooth number, size, morphology, structure, and location, are clinically significant in malocclusion, esthetics, and predisposing individuals to tooth caries and periodontal disorders in clinical manifestation [5]. Therefore, understanding dental abnormalities and differential diagnoses is critical for prompt management and appropriate intervention through clinical manifestation, female history, and hereditary pathways [6]. Radiography is used to distinguish missing teeth from impacted or embedded teeth, particularly those in the enamel and dentin complex and developmental anomalies include amelogenesis imperfecta, dentinogenesis imperfecta, dentin dysplasia [7]. More attention will be paid to developmental abnormalities in health society culture; reducing these anomalies requires regular dental care, a healthy diet, and excellent oral health habits. Dentists, pediatric dentists, orthodontists, and oral surgeons must be aware of abnormalities and use best practices for diagnosis and treatment, such as crowns, veneers, and tooth bonding, to maintain good oral hygiene. This chapter discusses current data focusing solely on enamel and dentin abnormalities, which phenotypical variable and difficult diagnosis in some cases and does not cover other dental anomalies, which allow specialists to diagnose and treat patients with amelogenesis imperfecta or dentinogenesis imperfecta in more recognizable ways.

## 2. Enamel and dentine abnormalities

The inadequate production of dentin and enamel, respectively, results in amelogenesis imperfecta and dentinogenesis imperfecta. Enamel and dentine abnormalities can cause disruptions to the structure of teeth due to hypoplasia, hypomineralization and hypomaturation in organic or inorganic components of the enamel and dentine. Hypoplasia and hypomineralization are common signs of developing enamel defects, whereas dentine abnormalities include dentine dysplasia and dentinogenesis imperfecta [8]. More often than not, the enamel defects present as anomalies of enamel and dentine with wearing, dentine-exposing and enamel cracks are regarded as clinical indicators and symptoms [9]. Sequences of enamel with dentine abnormalities increase endodontic issues due to dentine hypomineralization and pulp irregularities [10]. Due to data limitations, clinical evaluation of enamel defects is difficult. It entails reviewing the physical exams, imaging methods, and dental histories of patients. Gene mutations linked to DI and AI dysplasia, which impact tooth growth and shape, can be found through genetic testing. Tooth sample histological examination can shed light on the underlying reasons for anomalies in the enamel. Working together with pediatric dentists and geneticists can improve the precision and efficacy of clinical evaluations for identifying and treating anomalies in the enamel.

### 2.1 Amelogenesis imperfecta (AI)

Deviations in AI development include hypoplastic enamel, hypoplasia, hypomaturation, and hypocalcification, which increases susceptibility to caries, erosion, hypersensitivity, discoloration, and esthetic issues. AI may be linked to clinical dental conditions of other craniofacial abnormalities [11]. A delayed tooth eruption, an anterior open bite, pulp stones, taurodontism abnormalities are other dental conditions that may be linked to AI [12]. AI categories include genetic patterns and clinical and radiological criteria; Witkop [13] classified AI into four major types based on phenotype: hypoplastic, hypomaturation, hypocalcified and hypomaturation-hypoplastic [14]. Aldred and colleagues [15] also subclassified AI into four types (**Figure 1**) based on the future hereditary dental conditions that will be influenced by phenotype, including radiological, clinical, and other findings, as well as inheritance mode, molecular basis, and biochemical consequences [16]. Patients and specialists are familiar with the Witkop classification of amelogenesis imperfecta (AI) and will follow it in this context. Amelogenesis imperfecta (AI) is mostly caused by genetic abnormalities, whereby changes in genes with autosomal dominant or recessive inheritance patterns result in hypoplastic AI types and hypomature variations [17].

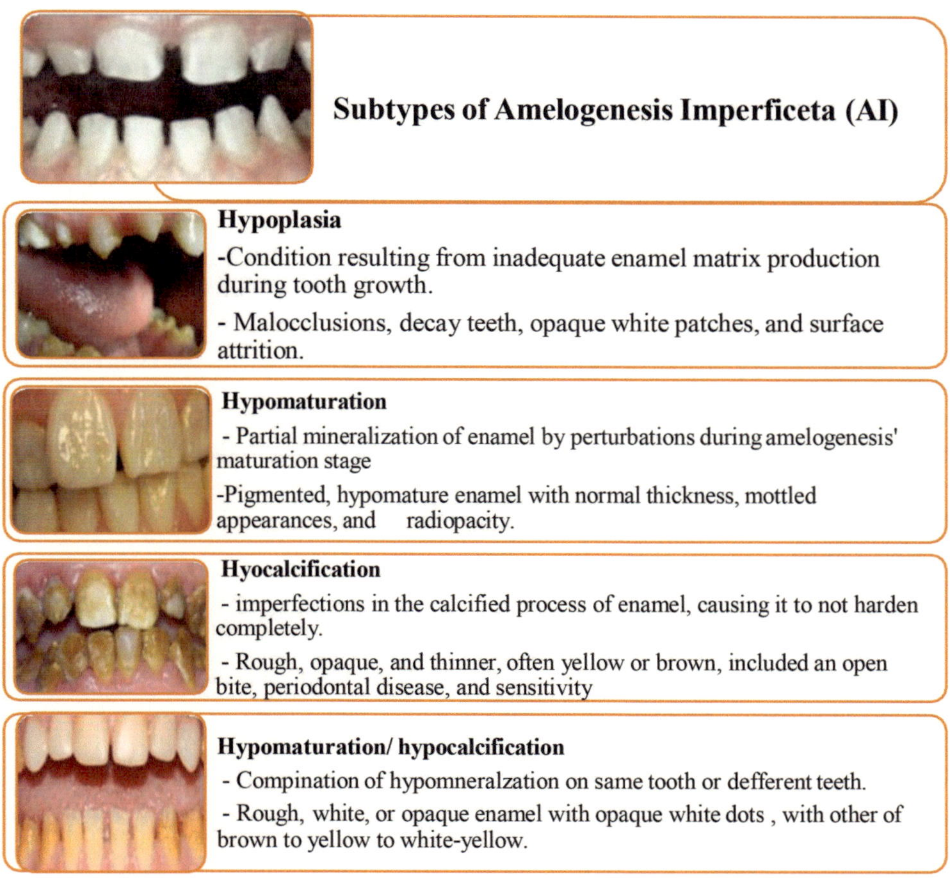


**Figure 1.**
*Clinical features of subtypes of Amelogenesis Imperfecta (AI).*

Acid phosphatase 4(ACP4) is the newly discovered gene known to be involved in hypocalcified autosomal dominant AI [18]. So far, there is different treatment plans among dentists on treat AI illness.

### *2.1.1 Hypoplasia AI type I*

Clinical signs of hypoplastic type 1 include decreased enamel thickness, malocclusions, many restorations, opaque white patches, and surface attrition. AI linked to enamel renal syndrome (ERS), a rare autosomal recessive condition characterized by thin enamel, late dental eruptions, intrapulpal calcifications, and bilateral nephrocalcinosis [15]. When compared to dentinogenesis hypoplastic, AI causes a reduction, radiopacity and enamel thickness. Large-scale genetics linked to syndromic types of AI should be included during the diagnostic process and taken into consideration as potential causes. Different genes and the inheritance can be either autosomal dominant or recessive, or X-linked. [14]. Heterozygous mutations in ENAM and LAMB3 genes can cause hypoplastic AI with markedly different phenotypes in Chinese patients [19]. It's important to note that although amelogenesis imperfecta (AI) subtypes can be linked to both autosomal recessive and autosomal dominant inheritance patterns, the autosomal dominant inheritance pattern (**Table 1**). In summary, thin or inadequate enamel, pits, or grooves on the surface of the teeth are signs of hypoplasia, which is caused by insufficient production of the enamel matrix during the growth of teeth.

### *2.1.2 Hypomaturation AI type II*

Hypomaturation AI type II is a condition characterized by pigmented, hypomature enamel with normal thickness, mottled appearances, and radiopacity. There is a lack of contrast between enamel and dentin, which is easily detached in families and potentially autosomal recessive subtyping [20]. Short stature syndrome, linked to gene mutations, associated with hypoplastic amelogenesis imperfecta is characterized by taurodontism, enamel hypoplasia, calcified dental pulp [21]. This condition is often linked to an open bite and enamel with a rough, creamy white to yellow-brown color that can be sensitive and painful (**Table 2**). Molar incisor hypomineralization (MIH) is a growing issue in children, causing hypomineralization on the first permanent molars and defined opacities. This can lead to caries due to teeth being fragile and prone to breaking. The exact cause is unknown, but factors such as environmental changes, nursing, respiratory conditions, low oxygen levels, and high-fever illnesses

| Subtype | Clinical Features | Genetic Basis |
|---|---|---|
| 1A | General, pitted rough enamels | Autosomal dominant |
| 1B | Local, pitted rough enamel, decays. | Autosomal dominant |
| IC | Local, pitted rough enamel | Autosomal recessive |
| ID | Diffuse, Smooth thin enamel | Autosomal dominant |
| IE | Diffuse, Smooth thin enamel | X-linked dominant |
| IF | Diffuse, Rough grooved enamel | autosomal dominant |
| IG | Enamel agenesis, complete / partial | autosomal recessive |

**Table 1.**
*Clinical features of subtypes of hypoplastic type 1.*

| Subtype | Clinical Features | Genetic Basis |
|---|---|---|
| IIA | Diffuse, pigmented, sensitive | Autosomal recessive |
| IIB | Diffuse, pigmented, rough teeth | Autosomal, recessive, X-linked |
| IIC | Snow-capped creamy, teeth | X- linked |
| IID | Snow-capped so white, teeth | Autosomal dominant |

**Table 2.**
*Clinical features of subtypes hypomaturation type II.*

are being researched [22]. MIH affects 3.6–39.3% of children and requires sensitive treatment. Treatment techniques include composite opaques, composite crown buildup, partial enamel removal, and micro abrasion. Dental caries is a risk factor for MIH, and sealants are effective for enamel restorations [23]. For extensive lesions or unresponsive sensitivity, full coronal coverage with stainless steel crowns is necessary. Radiographs showing bifurcation calcification should be used to assess the tooth's long-term survival [24]. Amelogenesis's maturity stage is when changes commonly occur that lead to hypocalcification, a disorder that causes incomplete mineralization of enamel, especially in teeth like molars and incisors. Enamel softening, staining, opacity, and greater susceptibility to decay are the characteristics of this disorder [25]. Teeth like these, either general or specialized, may be affected. Occasionally, genetic predispositions or certain medical conditions that affect the body's ability to properly mineralize enamel can lead to hypocalcification. A diet high in sugar and acid, along with poor oral hygiene practices, might make this issue worse.

### *2.1.3 Hypocalcified AI type III*

Hypocalcified AI type III was rough, opaque, and thinner, often yellow or brown. The patient's clinical features included an open bite, periodontal disease, and sensitivity (**Table 3**). Compared to the other subtypes, there are more teeth impacted in most of cases [26]. The radiograph revealed a reduction in enamel thickness and poorer radiopacity of the enamel in comparison to dentin [27]. AI type III is characterized by porous and soft enamel, leading to hypocalcification, discoloration, and increased wear sensitivity. This condition affects both primary and permanent teeth and can vary in severity, with some experiencing mild defects and others experiencing severe teeth prone to frequent cavities and breakage. Autosomal recessive inheritance is common in some cases.

### *2.1.4 Hypomaturation/hypocalcified with taurodontism AI type IV*

In one instance of this subtype, hypomaturation and hypocalcification traits are characterized by rough, white, or opaque enamel with opaque white dots.

| Subtype | Clinical Features | Genetic Basis |
|---|---|---|
| III A | General, pigmented | Autosomal dominant |
| III B | Local, pigmented | Autosomal, recessive |

**Table 3.**
*Clinical features of subtypes hypomaturation type III.*

| Subtype | Clinical Features | Genetic Basis |
|---|---|---|
| IVA | More hypomaturation with taurodontism | Autosomal dominant |
| | White spots, vertical lines, | |
| IVB | More hypocalcified, with taurodontism brown to yellow, or white to yellow | Autosomal, recessive |

**Table 4.**
*Clinical features of subtypes hypomaturation/hypocalcified type IV.*

Hypocalcification causes malocclusions, periodontal infections, and decreased enamel thickness (**Table 4**). Radiography shows radiopacity, enamel loss, and taurodontism in teeth [26]. The families in this subgroup displayed an autosomal recessive inheritance pattern. Rarely, hypomaturation and hypocalcification are present with diastemas, restorations, and susceptibility to temperature fluctuations Besides opaque, thin, and coarse enamel [27, 28]. Taurodontism is a dental anomaly caused by the apical displacement of the pulpal floor, an expanded pulp chamber, and a lack of constriction at the cemento-enamel junction. It is caused by Hertwig's epithelial root sheath's failure to invade [29]. Types of taurodontism include hypertaurodontism, mesotaurodontism, and hypotaurodontism, which vary in tooth size and shape relative to the dental arch, each with unique implications for dental health and function [30]. The most severe type causes root furcation at the root apices due to the larger pulp chamber and crown. In mild form, only the pulp chamber is expanded. Radiographic examination is used to identify taurodontism, with a prevalence rate ranging from 2.5 to 11.5%. Clinical problems may require different filling procedures and increase pulpal exposure risk due to the larger pulp chamber [31]. Mineral loss and deterioration in enamel are indicated by cavitations and pits, ranging from brown to yellow to white-yellow. These irregularities suggest poor oral hygiene and potential dental issues. Untreated pits and cavitations may worsen tooth sensitivity and decay. To prevent worsening oral health concerns, individuals with these surface irregularities should consult a dentist even in same cases mixed with different size of detention in terms of taurodontism.

## 2.2 Dentinogenesis imperfecta

Five categories of inherited dentin defects are recognized: two types of dentin dysplasia (DD) and three types of dentinogenesis imperfecta (DGI). Osteogenesis imperfecta (OGI) [32], a genetic condition causing bone diseases, occurs through mutations in two genes that encode type I collagen fiber formation, always linked with two type of DD and DGI [33]. Dentin sialophosphoprotein (DSPP) mutations cause other various types of dentinogenetic defects, each with a unique inherited pattern in dentition [34]. The genetic revolution has not affected the rare DD-I subtype, which has short, blunt roots and obliterated pulp chambers and whose etiology is currently unknown [35]. Generally, dentinogenesis imperfecta and dentine dysplasia affecting dentin formation, resulting in altered dentin morphology across all teeth (**Figure 2**). There are three main kinds of dentinogenesis imperfecta, which affect dentin formation and cause changes in morphology in all teeth (**Table 5**). Type I (DGI-I): Osteogenesis imperfecta is associated with symptoms in the teeth structural defects DGI-I [36]. Type II (DGI-II): traditional hereditary opalescent dentine that has clinical, radiological, and histological characteristics similar to DGI Type I but lacks impaired osteogenesis. Type III (DGI-III): Brandywine isolate is opalescent dentine that has been specifically isolated from the Brandywine region of Maryland. mutations in a number of genes, including DSPP,

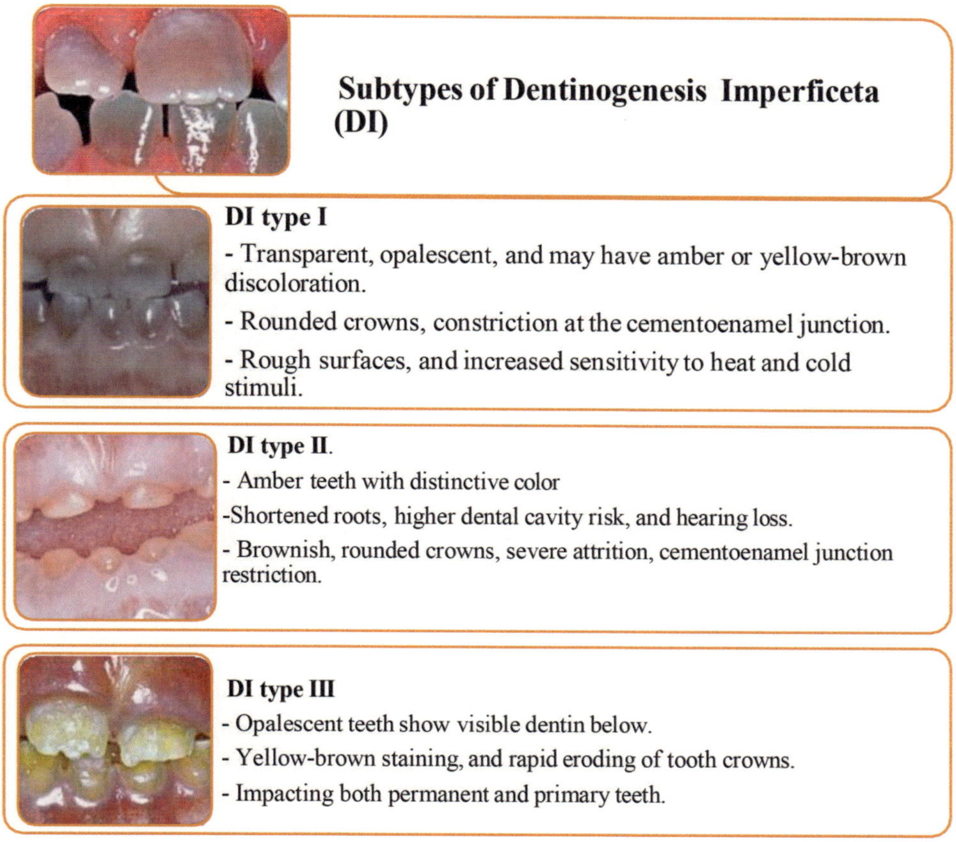


**Figure 2.**
*Clinical features of subtypes of Dentinogenesis Imperfecta (DI).*

| Subtype | Clinical Features | Genetic Basis |
|---|---|---|
| DGI-I with osteogenesis imperfecta | Blue-gray to yellow-brown teeth, enamel fracturing, excessive wear primary teeth more affected than permanent. (occurs as clinical feature of osteogenesis imperfecta), bulbous crown | Mutations of collagen type 1(genes (COLIAI &II) |
| DGI-II without osteogenesis imperfecta | Pulp obliteration which differentiates between type I & II, Similar to DI-I More severe in permanent more than primary dentitions, irregular crowns. | Commonly, linked to 4921 Locus |
| DGI-III | Similar clinically to type I & II expressed with enamel wearing and attrition to gingival level. There is a large pulp, thin dentin, bulbus grown. | Probably, linked to 4921 Locus |

**Table 5.**
*Clinical features of three types of dentinogenesis imperfecta.*

COL1A1, and COL1A2 [37]. In summary, Dentinogenesis imperfecta is hereditary and genetic in nature and is characterized by abnormalities in dentin formation, leading to fragile, discolored, and wear-prone teeth. It affects both permanent and deciduous dentition, with deciduous teeth being more severely affected. This shed light on the clinical features and genetic basis of each subtype of dentinogenesis imperfecta.

### *2.2.1 Dentinogenesis imperfecta type I (DGI-I)*

Dentinogenesis imperfecta type I (DI-I), is inherited in an autosomal dominant manner as clinical sign of systemic osteogenesis imperfecta. It leads to complex clinical symptoms like pulp obliteration, opalescent brown, tooth wear, and attrition, and is also present in Goldblatt syndromes and Ehlers-Danlos syndromes [38]. It affects both permanent and deciduous dentition and is brought on by mutations in the procollagen type I COL1A1 or COL1A2 gene as in similarity to osteogenesis imperfecta [39]. DGI-I patients have genetic defects that disrupt collagen fibril development in teeth's dentin, affecting their strength and appearance, resulting in altered dentinal tubule shape, fewer tubules, and smaller widths [40]. The genetic bone-brittle condition known as osteogenesis imperfecta is accompanied by dentinogenesis imperfecta. It is brought on by gene mutations that code for type I collagen, the substance that gives bones their strength [41]. There are different types, but the most common and moderate type is OGI-I. The probability of acquiring OGI is higher in families where the disorder has a history. Individuals with DI-I may experience dental pain and increased sensitivity to hot or cold temperatures. The pre- and post-treatment plans for oral hygiene and rehabilitation are part of the management of dentinogenesis imperfecta (DGI-I) as crowns and restorations are included.

### *2.2.2 Dentinogenesis imperfecta type II (DGI-II)*

Dentinogenesis imperfecta (DGI-II) is an autosomal dominant disorder with clinical and radiological characteristics similar to type I. It has short, constricted roots, opalescent teeth, and soft, blue-brown, transparent teeth [42]. Primary and secondary dentitions have structural irregularities, causing pulp obliteration, which acts as second base to differentiate between type I and II [43]. The DSPP gene, found on chromosome 4q22.1, acts as gene basis mutation of the condition [44]. Bulbous crowns, cervical constriction, and osteogenesis are common, and hearing loss may occur. The degree of symptoms and the demands of the patient determine the treatment options for hereditary dental problems. Frequent check-ups with a dental staff are essential for required modifications.

### *2.2.3 Dentinogenesis imperfecta type III (DGI-III)*

Dentinogenesis imperfecta type III, also known as the "Brandywine" variety, is an uncommon disorder affecting the Brandywine community in Maryland, USA. The DSPP gene produces dental sialoprotein, dental glycoprotein, and dental phosphoprotein, all derived from the dentin matrix [45]. The DSPP gene can result in reduced DSPP protein, incorrect calcification, insufficient dentin mineralization, or accumulation in odontoblasts, impacting protein processing and transport during dentin matrix formation [46]. When dentine production stops after the mantle layer forms, multiple pulpal exposures occur in the primary dentition, giving teeth the radiographic appearance of shell teeth.

## 2.3 Dentine dysplasia

Dentine dysplasia is a condition where teeth lack roots, with symptoms like pulpal obliteration, periapical radiolucency, and short or absent roots (**Figure 3**). It can be classified into two types: type I, known as radicular dentine dysplasia, where roots are

*DOI: http://dx.doi.org/10.5772/intechopen.114134*

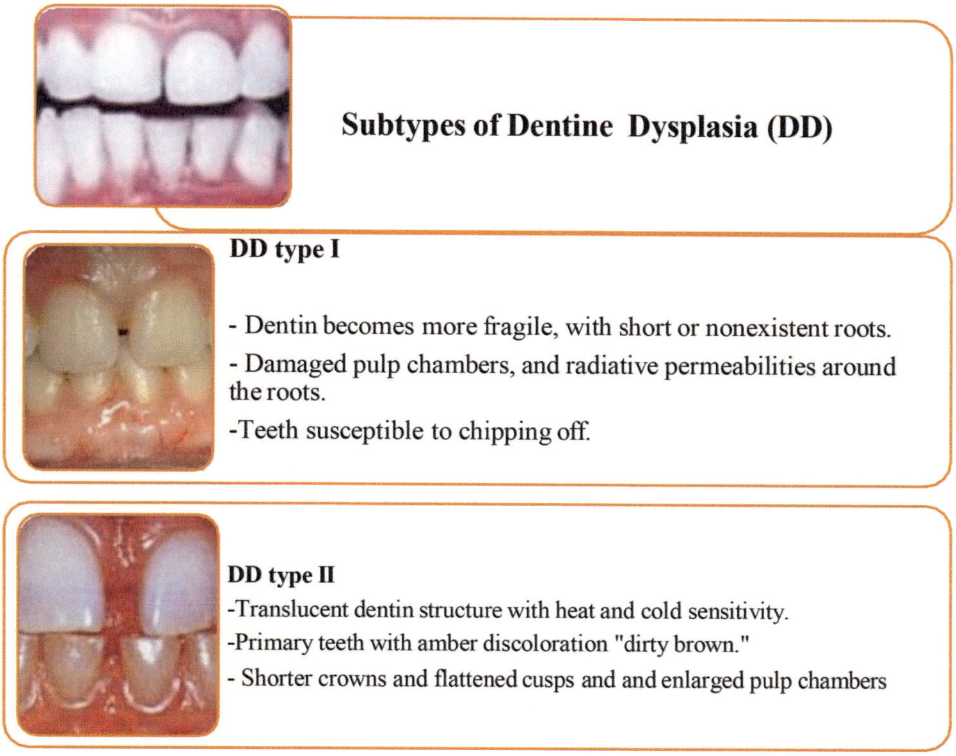


**Figure 3.**
*Clinical features of subtypes of dentine dysplasia (DD).*

completely absent, and type II, also known as coronal dentine dysplasia, with short or malformed roots (**Table 6**). Dentine dysplasia is a rare hereditary condition affecting 1% of permanent and 1% of deciduous teeth [47]. It causes dental anomalies like radiolucent lesions, undeveloped roots, enlarged pulp chambers, and premature tooth loss. The SIBLING family, consisting of dentin and sialophosphoprotein (DSPP), is involved in producing defects like DSP, DGP, and DPP [48]. Its clinical feature similar to dentinogenesis imperfecta, to control symptoms and improve oral health, specific dental treatments may be needed. The condition is distinguished by aberrant dentin production, resulting in short roots, radiolucency, and early exfoliation.

### *2.3.1 Dentine dysplasia type I (DD-I)*

It is an uncommon disorder, likely an allelic condition of the DSPP gene, that causes small crowns in primary and permanent dentitions, smaller crescentic pulps,

| Subtype | Clinical Features | Genetic Basis |
|---|---|---|
| DD-I | Misaligned teeth, permanent teeth have normal to slight blue gray color, | Unknown, |
| DD-II | dentin frequent absent in primary teeth. Pulp obliteration in both primary or permanent teeth | Unknown |

**Table 6.**
*Clinical features of dentine dysplasia subtypes.*

and periapical radiolucency. It results in abnormal tooth dentine development, making weakened teeth prone to decay and breakage. Type I dentin dysplasia, also known as DD-I, is a rare genetic disorder that affects the development of dentin, the hard tissue that forms the majority of a tooth [49]. It is characterized by short, conical, pointed roots or teeth without roots, impacting both primary and permanent dentition with minor frequency of DD-I is estimated to be 1/100,000 [50]. This condition can result in weakened teeth that are prone to fractures and premature loss.

#### *2.3.2 Dentine dysplasia type II (DD-II)*

It is a minor form of dentinogenesis abnormalities, characterized by clinically normal permanent teeth with a thistle-shaped pulp and stones, and no periapical radiolucency. It is caused by a mutation in the DSPP gene and is a less severe form of type I dentine dysplasia [51]. Dentin dysplasia type II, also known as coronal dentin dysplasia, is a rare genetic condition affecting dentin formation. Clinically, causing brownish-blue staining teeth and pulp destruction.

## 3. Conclusion

Abnormalities in the enamel-dentine can lead to cavities, attrition, erosion, cosmetic issues, and tooth sensitivity, which can be inherited. A balanced diet, regular dental care, and good oral hygiene practices are essential for preserving tooth structure and enhancing function. Early identification and management are critical for these outcomes. Dentine dysplasia can be difficult to diagnose and treat and can cause orthodontic and endodontic treatment failure. Dentists, pediatric dentists, orthodontists, and oral surgeons must be aware of these abnormalities and adhere to best practices, considering genetic variables and family history.

## Acknowledgements

I would like to express my gratitude to associate professor M.E. Önger for his encouragement and help during the figure's preparation processes. My profound appreciation to the manager of Ondokuz Mayis University's teaching dentistry hospital.

## Conflict of interest

The authors declare no conflict of interest.

## Appendices and nomenclature

| | |
|---|---|
| AI | amelogenesis imperfecta |
| DI | dentinogenesis imperfecta |
| DD | dentine dysplasia |
| DSPP | dentine sialophosphoprotein |
| MIH | molar-incisor hypomineralization |

| | |
|---|---|
| DGI | dentinogenesis imperfecta |
| OGI | osteogenesis imperfecta |
| CPP-ACP | calcium phosphopeptide-amorphous calcium phosphate |
| DSP | dentine sialoprotein |
| DGP | dentinogenesis protein |
| DPP | dentine phosphoprotein |

## Author details

Abubaker El Elhaj
Ondokuz Mayis University, Samsun, Turkey

*Address all correspondence to: abubaker.elhaj@omu.edu.tr;
abubakerelhaj@gmail.com

## References

[1] Costa FS et al. Developmental defects of enamel and dental caries in the primary dentition: A systematic review and meta-analysis. Journal of Dentistry. 2017;**60**:1-7. DOI: 10.1016/j. j.dent.2017.03.006

[2] Torlińska-Walkowiak N et al. Developmental enamel defects and dental anomalies of number and size in children with growth hormone deficiency. Scientific Reports. 2023;**13**(1):14707. DOI: 10.1038/s41598-023-41892-x

[3] Liang T et al. Mutant dentin sialophosphoprotein causes dentinogenesis imperfecta. Journal of Dental Research. 2019;**98**(8):912-919. DOI: 10.1177/0022034519854029

[4] Rohilla M. Etiology of various dental developmental anomalies-review of literature. Journal of Dental Problems and Solutions. 2017;**4**(2):19-25. DOI: 10.17352/2394-8418.000042

[5] Koch G, Thesleff I, Kreiborg S. Tooth development and disturbances in number and shape of teeth. Pediatric Dentistry: A Clinical Approach. Wiley, google books; 2017. p. 3

[6] Flaitz CM. Differential diagnosis of oral lesions and developmental anomalies. In: Pediatric Dentistry. Elsevier, Science Direct; 2019. pp. 8-49. e1

[7] Kühnisch J et al. Best clinical practice guidance for prescribing dental radiographs in children and adolescents: An EAPD policy document. European Archives of Pediatric Dentistry. 2020;**21**:375-386. DOI: 10.1007/s40368-019-00493-x

[8] Sawan NM. Clear aligners in patients with amelogenesis and dentinogenesis imperfecta. International Journal of Dentistry. 2021;**2021**:7343094. DOI: 10.1155/2021/7343094

[9] Grande F, Catapano S. Developmental dental defects and tooth wear: Pathological processes relationship. In: Human Tooth and Developmental Dental Defects-Compositional and Genetic Implications. Intech Open; 2021. DOI: 10.5772/intechopen.99420

[10] Sabandal MM, Dammaschke T, Schäfer E. Restorative treatment in a case of amelogenesis imperfecta and 9-year follow-up: A case report. Head & Face Medicine. 2020;**16**(1):1-8. DOI: 10.1186/s13005-020-00243-1

[11] Ceyhan D, Kirzioglu Z, Emek T. A long-term clinical study on individuals with amelogenesis imperfecta. Nigerian Journal of Clinical Practice. 2019;**22**(8):1157-1162. DOI: 10.4103/njcp.njcp_227_18

[12] Wimalarathna A et al. Amelogenesis imperfecta: A literature review-based guide to diagnosis and management. Journal of Multidisciplinary Dentistry. 2020;**10**(3):94-101. DOI: 10.46875/jmd.v10i3.532

[13] Witkop C, Jr. Amelogenesis imperfecta, dentinogenesis imperfecta and dentin dysplasia revisited: Problems in classification. Journal of Oral Pathology. 1988;**17**:547-553

[14] Toupenay S et al. Amelogenesis imperfecta: Therapeutic strategy from primary to permanent dentition across case reports. BMC Oral Health. 2018;**18**(1):1-8. DOI: 10.1186/s12903-018-0554-y

[15] Aldred M, Savarirayan R, Crawford P. Amelogenesis imperfecta: A

classification and catalogue for the 21st century. Oral Diseases. 2003;**9**(1):19-23. DOI: 10.1034/j.1601-0825.2003.00843.x

[16] Appelstrand S, Robertson A, Sabel N. Patient-reported outcome measures in individuals with amelogenesis imperfecta: A systematic review. European Archives of Paediatric Dentistry. 2022;**23**(6):885-895. DOI: 10.1007/s40368-022-00737-3

[17] Lu T et al. Whole exome sequencing identifies an AMBN missense mutation causing severe autosomal-dominant amelogenesis imperfecta and dentin disorders. International Journal of Oral Science. 2018;**10**(3):26. DOI: 10.1038/s41368-018-0027-9

[18] Kim YJ et al. Recessive mutations in ACP4 cause amelogenesis imperfecta. Journal of Dental Research. 2022;**101**(1):37-45. DOI: 10.1177/00220345211015119

[19] Wang X et al. Novel ENAM and LAMB3 mutations in Chinese families with hypoplastic amelogenesis imperfecta. PLoS One. 2015;**10**(3):e0116514. DOI: 10.1371/journal.pone.0116514

[20] Nouara F et al. First characterization of LTBP3 variants in two Moroccan families with hypoplastic amelogenesis imperfecta. Archives of Oral Biology. 2022;**142**:105518. DOI: 10.1016/j.archoralbio.2022.105518

[21] Kantaputra P et al. Expanding genotypic and phenotypic spectrums of LTBP3 variants in dental anomalies and short stature syndrome. Clinical Genetics. 2022;**102**(1):66-71. DOI: 10.1111/cge.14134

[22] Rodd HD et al. Molar incisor hypomineralization: Current knowledge and practice. International Dental Journal. 2021;**71**(4):285-291. DOI: 10.1111/idj.12624

[23] Somani C et al. An update of treatment modalities in children and adolescents with teeth affected by molar incisor hypomineralization (MIH): A systematic review. European Archives of Pediatric Dentistry. 2022;**23**(1):39-64. DOI: 10.1007/s40368-021-00635-0

[24] Mathew MG et al. Evaluation of clinical success, parental and child satisfaction of stainless-steel crowns and zirconia crowns in primary molars. Journal of Family Medicine and Primary Care. 2020;**9**(3):1418. DOI: 10.4103/jfmpc.jfmpc_1006_19

[25] Siddiqui S, Saba I. Demineralization and Remineralization of Teeth. Edu Bubs Publishing House google books.com; 2020

[26] Lundgren GP et al. Experiences of being a parent to a child with amelogenesis imperfecta. Dentistry Journal. 2019;**7**(1):17. DOI: 10.3390/dj7010017

[27] Adorno-Farias D et al. Diversity of clinical, radiographic and genealogical findings in 41 families with amelogenesis imperfecta. Journal of Applied Oral Science. 2019;**27**:e20180359. DOI: 10.1590/1678-7757-2018-0359

[28] Kotsanos N et al. Developmental defects of the teeth and their hard tissues. In: Pediatric Dentistry. Springer International Publishing; 2022. pp. 415-463. DOI: 10.1007/978-3-030-78003-6_17

[29] Yamamoto T et al. Hertwig's epithelial root sheath fate during initial cellular cementogenesis in rat molars. Acta Histochemica et Cytochemica. 2015;**48**(3):95-101. DOI: 10.1267/ahc.15006

[30] Chetty M, Roomaney IA, Beighton P. Taurodontism in dental genetics. BDJ open. 2021;**7**(1):25. DOI: 10.1038/s41405-021-00081-6

[31] Samji ZB. Investigating the Prevalence of Taurodontism in an Adolescent Population Using Dental Panoramic Radiographs. University of British Columbia; 2021. DOI: 10.14288/1.0400885

[32] Kaur S, et al. Design, synthesis and evaluation of benzimidazole hybrids to inhibit acetylcholinesterase and COX for treatment of Alzheimer's disease. Central Nervous System Agents in Medicinal Chemistry (Formerly Current Medicinal Chemistry-Central Nervous System Agents). 2022;**22**(1):68-78. DOI: 10.2174/1871524922666220428134001

[33] Su T et al. Hereditary dentin defects with systemic diseases. Oral Diseases. 2023;**29**(6):2376-2393. DOI: 10.1111/odi.14589

[34] Liu M et al. Dentine sialophosphoprotein signal in dentinogenesis and dentine regeneration. European Cells & Materials. 2021;**42**:43. DOI: 10.22203/eCM.v042a04

[35] Putrino A et al. Type I dentin dysplasia: The literature review and case report of a family affected by misrecognition and late diagnosis. Medicina. 2023;**59**(8):1477. DOI: 10.3390/medicina59081477

[36] Ibrahim S et al. Phenotypic properties of collagen in dentinogenesis imperfecta associated with osteogenesis imperfecta. International Journal of Nanomedicine. 2019;**14**:9423-9435. DOI: 10.2147/IJN.S217420

[37] Nutchoey O et al. Phenotypic features of dentinogenesis imperfecta associated with osteogenesis imperfecta and COL1A2 mutations. Oral Surgery, Oral Medicine, Oral Pathology and Oral Radiology. 2021;**131**(6):694-701. DOI: 10.1016/j.oooo.2021.01.003

[38] Kapferer-Seebacher I et al. Dental manifestations of Ehlers-Danlos syndromes: A systematic review. Acta Dermato-Venereologica. 2020;**100**(7):152-160. DOI: 10.2340/00015555-3428

[39] Tournis S, Dede AD. Osteogenesis imperfecta–a clinical update. Metabolism. 2018;**80**:27-37. DOI: 10.1016/j.metabol.2017.06.001

[40] Carreon AH, Funkenbusch PD. Nanoscale properties and deformation of human enamel and dentin. Journal of the Mechanical Behavior of Biomedical Materials. 2019;**97**:74-84. DOI: 10.1016/j.jmbbm.2019.05.009

[41] Gama FJR et al. Dentinogenesis imperfecta type II: A case report with 17 years of follow-up. Imaging Science in Dentistry. 2017;**47**(2):129-133. DOI: 10.5624/isd.2017.47.2.129

[42] Garrocho-Rangel A et al. Dentinogenesis imperfecta type II in children: A scoping review. Journal of Clinical Pediatric Dentistry. 2019;**43**(3):147-154. DOI: 10.17796/1053-4625-43.3.1

[43] Andersson K et al. Dentinogenesis imperfecta type II in Swedish children and adolescents. Orphanet Journal of Rare Diseases. 2018;**13**:1-7. DOI: 10.1186/s13023-018-0887-2

[44] Porntaveetus T et al. Compromised alveolar bone cells in a patient with dentinogenesis imperfecta caused by DSPP mutation. Clinical Oral Investigations. 2019;**23**:303-313. DOI: 10.1007/s00784-018-2437-7

[45] Yamakoshi Y, Simmer JP. Structural features, processing mechanism

and gene splice variants of dentin sialophosphoprotein. Japanese Dental Science Review. 2018;**54**(4):183-196. DOI: 10.1016/j.jdsr.2018.03.006

[46] Liu M et al. BMP signaling pathway in dentin development and diseases. Cell. 2022;**11**(14):2216. DOI: 10.3390/cells11142216

[47] Ye X et al. Dentin dysplasia type I—Novel findings in deciduous and permanent teeth. BMC Oral Health. 2015;**15**(1):1-9. DOI: 10.1186/s12903-015-0149-9

[48] Liang T et al. Enamel defects associated with dentin sialophosphoprotein mutation in mice. Frontiers in Physiology. 2021;**12**:724098. DOI: 10.3389/fphys.2021.724098

[49] Chen D et al. Dentin dysplasia type I—A dental disease with genetic heterogeneity. Oral Diseases. 2019;**25**(2):439-446. DOI: 10.1111/odi.12861

[50] Severin E, Moldoveanu GG, Moldoveanu A. Failure of tooth development: Prevalence, genetic causes and clinical features. In: Human Tooth and Developmental Dental Defects-Compositional and Genetic Implications. Intech Open Books; 2021. DOI: 10.5772/intechopen.99419

[51] Liang T et al. Dentin defects caused by a Dspp− 1 frameshift mutation are associated with the activation of autophagy. Scientific Reports. 2023;**13**(1):6393. DOI: 10.1038/s41598-023-33362-1

Chapter 4

# Advancements in Preventive Strategies and Enamel Regeneration: Navigating the Complexities of Dental Care in the Age of Technology

*Atena Galuscan, Daniela Jumanca and Ramona Dumitrescu*

## Abstract

In our technology-driven world, rising dental injuries have prompted re-evaluation of treatment methods. Key focuses include preventing carious lesions through early detection and good oral hygiene. Precise diagnostic tools enable tailored treatments, such as fluoridation, sealing, pH-adjusting diets, resin infiltration, and ozone remineralization. Dental enamel is crucial for tooth function. Researchers aim to replicate its complex structure for biocompatible materials. Hydroxyapatite's unique properties are vital for hard tissues like bones, enamel, and dentin. Enamel development involves ameloblasts in pre-eruptive and post-eruptive stages. Saliva aids post-eruptive maturation but can lead to bacterial adhesion and enamel demineralization. Preventing enamel demineralization hinges on ion transport and critical pH levels, while low calcium levels impact enamel cells. Dietary sugars interact with bacteria, causing demineralization, but saliva aids remineralization. Caries risk depends on factors like diet, oral hygiene, and tooth morphology. Personalized approaches like Caries Management by Risk Assessment (CAMBRA) for caries risk assessment (CRA) are crucial. Traditional enamel protection methods involve fluoride and dental sealants, but concerns exist about fluoride toxicity and bacterial resistance. Modern alternatives include resin infiltration for early caries, argon laser technique for lesion protection, and ozone therapy to combat decay, offering noninvasive options for enamel care.

**Keywords:** preventable disease, carious lesions, enamel remineralization, sealing techniques, saliva's properties

## 1. Introduction

We find ourselves in an era characterized by rapid technological advancements, unlike any other time in history. However, despite this progress, we continue to grapple with an alarming increase in dental injuries across all age groups. This contemporary predicament raises questions about the effectiveness of our current treatment approaches and the validity of our problem-solving strategies.

Within the realm of medical science, carious lesions are officially recognized as a disease, aptly named carious disease. Consequently, it's crucial to acknowledge that, unlike many other health conditions, carious lesions are preventable. To stave off the development of carious lesions, it becomes imperative to diligently assess the risk of tooth decay and identify demineralization lesions in their early stages. Furthermore, it is essential to formulate and implement the most efficient preventive measures.

To this day, the most renowned method for averting cavities remains fluoridation. Over time, this practice has persisted and is still applied through various means such as gels, varnishes, mouthwashes, and toothpaste formulations. A secondary preventive approach entails sealing fissures and gaps with sealing materials, including resins and ionomer-based cements.

However, in addition to these major preventive techniques, the maintenance of oral hygiene plays a pivotal role in ensuring the success of these methods. Moreover, the dietary habits of the individual can either bolster or undermine the effectiveness of the aforementioned therapies. Daily consumption of carbohydrates and sugars in various forms causes a decline in salivary pH levels, exposing tooth enamel to recurrent acid attacks, resulting in the development of demineralization lesions.

Hence, the effectiveness of any preventive strategy against carious lesions hinges on imparting health education regarding nutrition and oral hygiene to induce a transformation in patient behavior and lifestyle. This underscores the idea that dental issues are not contagious but rather stem from individual behaviors.

Consequently, the management of enamel quality should initiate with the identification and regulation of individual-level risk factors, followed by education on sound dietary choices and dental hygiene practices. Subsequently, non-invasive preventive enamel treatments can be considered.

Regarding these treatments, the approach must be distinctive. To select the most suitable therapy, accurate diagnosis by the dentist is essential. Various medical instruments, such as intraoral cameras, Diagnodent, VistaCam iX, or the office version of CLMS, facilitate this precise diagnosis.

Following a meticulous examination and diagnosis, the appropriate treatment can be determined, which may involve fluoridation, sealing, dietary adjustments to elevate salivary pH, infiltration using low-viscosity resins, or Ozone remineralization (O3T).

### 1.1 Enamel: understanding the structure and characteristics of dental enamel

The outermost layer of a tooth is composed of dental enamel, making it the hardest tissue in the human body. Conversely, the innermost part of the tooth is occupied by the dental pulp, a crucial component housing specialized cells, nerves, and blood vessels. The dental pulp, in conjunction with dentin, constitutes the pulpo-dental organ, playing a vital role in preserving the tooth's vitality [1].

It directly enables and powers the mechanical processes of cutting, breaking, and grinding, making its mechanical characteristics highly impressive [2]. These attributes result from the flawless realization of the prismatic spatial microstructure of hydroxyapatite. Enamel's exceptional mineralization as a cellular tissue is attributed to its composition, comprising 97% inorganic matter, 3% organic matter, and 1% water.

Over the past few years, experts in the dental materials and dental medicine field have been striving to replicate a biomimetic enamel-like structure possessing identical mechanical characteristics [3]. Innovative methods, including surfactant-assisted techniques, hydrogel systems, and high-temperature, high-pressure hydrothermal systems, have even been employed to endeavor the regeneration of hydroxyapatite (HA) crystals [3].

Replicating the *in vitro* biomechanical traits of enamel poses a challenge due to their intricate nature, stemming from the hierarchical organization of enamel prisms across multiple tiers. These prismatic frameworks are intricately interwoven and closely knit, comprising hydroxyapatite (HA) crystals aligned in parallel [4]. Research has indicated that dental synthetic materials designed to mimic enamel-like structures exhibit superior biocompatibility when compared to materials with randomly arranged structures [4]. As a result, it is imperative, in the pursuit of materials for promoting enamel remineralization, to faithfully replicate the prism structure found in dental enamel [5].

The distinctive microstructure of enamel extends perpendicularly from the enamel-dentin junction to the enamel surface [6], resulting in anisotropic mechanical properties [6]. Research has quantified enamel hardness through Young's moduli measurements, revealing values in the range of 85–90 GPa parallel to the crystalline rod axis and 70–77 GPa perpendicular to it. The average hardness registers at approximately 4.79 GPa parallel to the enamel rods and 3.8 GPa perpendicular to them, with a hardness of approximately 0.7 ± 0.02 MPa*m^1/2 [5, 7].

### 1.2 Exploring the world of hydroxyapatite ($Ca10(PO_4)_6{\cdot}2(OH)$)

Hydroxyapatite is a fundamental component found not only in the hard tissues of the human body but also in various other structures. In the skeletal system, for instance, it constitutes 65% of its composition, playing a critical role in conferring rigidity and strength to bones. Additionally, HA holds a central position as the primary mineral component in both enamel and dentin [8].

Literature studies have indicated that in enamel, HA crystals typically range in size from 48 to 78 nm [8]. These crystals exhibit a hexagonal shape and collectively form rod-like structures within the enamel, in contrast to the flattened rods found in mature dentin, which measure approximately 60–70 nm in length [9].

The remarkable stability and low solubility of HA in nature can be attributed to its calcium-phosphorus ratio of 1:67 [9]. Over time, owing to its exceptional properties, the calcium-phosphorus system has garnered significant attention in medical research, finding applications in fields such as implantology, the skeletal system, and drug delivery systems [10].

### 1.3 Delving into enamel mineralization

Describing the intricacies of enamel development and maturation is a formidable task. This process, in terms of its duration, can be likened to the gestation of an embryo within the womb, but it unfolds over a considerably longer period than enamel amelogenesis [1]. Achieving full maturity in the crown formation of specific permanent teeth may even span up to 5 years [1]. Once maturity is attained, dental enamel comprises a substantial 95% of its weight in hydroxyapatite crystals [1].

A diverse assembly of specialized cells [11] contributes to the formation of enamel. Collaboration among these cells, both intercellular and with the surrounding tissues, is a noteworthy aspect of this process, involving transformative elements with distinct functions [11–13].

Among these cells, ameloblasts hold the utmost significance. These tall and columnar epithelial cells, characterized by structures like the "Tomes process" [14, 15], bear the responsibility for both mineralizing and shaping enamel [11].

Furthermore, the developmental islands play a pivotal role in facilitating proper enamel development. Enamel, being an acellular organ, lacks the capacity for remodeling once it undergoes mineralization [11]. Enamel development is a multifaceted process comprised of two distinct stages: the pre-eruptive and post-eruptive phases. In the initial stage, mineralization is orchestrated by pre-eruptive cells. Here, ameloblasts play a central role in directing the synthesis of matrix proteins and commencing the formation of enamel crystals [1].

The process of amelogenesis at this level unfolds in two developmental phases: secretory and maturation. In the secretory phase, ameloblasts initiate the release of matrix proteins from the enamel and commence their outward migration from the enamel organ [16, 17].

Within the secretory stage, four distinct cell layers are discernible: an inner layer of secretory ameloblasts, an intermediate zone comprising one or two layers of slender cells, the stellate reticulum layer, and an outer layer forming the enamel's outer epithelium [18, 19]. The vascular network responsible for supplying essential nutrients during enamel development circulates and interacts with the outer epithelial layer of the enamel [18, 19].

Ameloblasts hold particular significance in this context as they synthesize four primary structural proteins and two proteases (metalloprotease 20—MMP20—and Kallikrein 4) that collectively contribute to the shaping and spatial organization of the initial hydroxyapatite (HA) [14, 15].

Among the four principal structural proteins, *amelogenin* takes precedence. It is the most abundantly secreted and plays a pivotal role in the growth and organization of the enamel structure, governing its morphology [20]. As an intrinsically disordered protein, amelogenin assumes a crucial role in controlling the polymorphism of calcium phosphate [21, 22].

The second enamel protein is ameloblastin. While its exact function remains to be fully elucidated, it is believed to be indispensable for enamel formation [1]. Enamelin, though present in the least quantity, is consistently found at all stages during enamel formation [1] and collaborates with amelogenin with a strong affinity for apatite crystals [23].

The fourth protein in this lineup is amelotin, and its exact role remains a mystery; what's clear is that it is secreted by maturing ameloblasts. These proteins are distributed in various locations within the enamel, underscoring their vital role in enamel development [24]. In the inner enamel layer, these proteins are found in fragments, while in the outer layer, intact protein molecules are prevalent [24].

During the maturation stage, there's a notable shift in ameloblast function, transitioning from a secretory role to one integral to the mineralization process [25]. They reconfigure themselves to assume the responsibility of calcium transport [1, 26], a function of paramount importance during the maturation phase. Any disruption in calcium transport can result in incomplete enamel mineralization [13].

Kallikrein 4 (kallikrein-related peptidase 4 (KLK4)) also plays a crucial role, as it breaks down proteins in the enamel matrix. This enzymatic degradation by KLK4 creates space for the expansion of mineral crystals [1]. Following this degradation, ameloblasts absorb the smaller fragments, which are subsequently broken down by lysosomes [1].

After a tooth's eruption, it exhibits a layer of enamel covered by an enamel film [27]. In this post-eruptive maturation stage, the primary role shifts to saliva, as it facilitates the diffusion of calcium, phosphorus, potassium, magnesium, and fluoride ions to the enamel surface through interaction with saliva [27].

While the salivary film aids in the post-eruptive maturation stage of enamel, it can also potentially contribute to bacterial adhesion, potentially leading to enamel demineralization and the development of carious lesions [1, 27].

### 1.4 Understanding enamel demineralization

The formation of enamel crystallites is heavily influenced by ion transport, particularly involving $Ca^{2+}$ and $PO_4$ 3 ions [5]. These ions are transported into the enamel matrix, leading to changes in the $Ca/PO_4$ ratio within the calcified enamel matrix [5].

In systems with cation-selective membranes, crystal growth results in an increased length/width ratio, a decreased width/thickness ratio, and elevated $Ca^{2+}$ and $PO_4$ concentrations [13]. For instance, $H^+$ ions play a crucial role in promoting crystal growth in the longitudinal direction [5].

When crystal growth occurs in membranes with lower pH values and reduced $PO_4$ concentrations, it tends to exhibit preferential growth in the c-axis direction [5].

Regarding enamel demineralization, the focus shifts to pH levels, as hydroxy-apatite dissolution is enhanced with decreasing pH and the concentrations of $Ca^{2+}$, $PO_4^{3-}$ (and OH-) in the solution [28]. The degree of saturation concerning HA (DS HA) is defined as the ratio of the product of the ionic activity for HA to the solubility constant for HA, known as K-HA [28].

The crucial point at which pH decreases significantly is referred to as the "pH-critical" point, signifying the pH level at which a solution reaches saturation concerning a particular mineral. At this juncture, dental enamel exists in equilibrium, with neither dissolution nor precipitation of minerals occurring [28]. The critical pH for enamel is now widely accepted to be between 4.5 and 5.5 [29].

The degree of saturation (DS) of the plaque solution in relation to polycyclic aromatic hydrocarbons (PAH) plays a central role in influencing the rate of tooth demineralization [30]. This is predominantly determined by the pH value and the concentrations of calcium and hydrogen phosphate ions.

A sharp decline in pH is immediately associated with a reduction in DS, leading to a sudden escalation in the demineralization rate and subsequently an increase in calcium ion concentration [30].

When the pH falls below a critical threshold, the system becomes undersaturated, significantly heightening the potential for enamel demineralization [28].

Numerous studies are underway to explore the factors influencing the critical pH and enamel dissolution [31]. For instance, the concentrations of calcium and phosphate in saliva, particularly in contact with enamel, can impact the degree of saturation. According to mechanical *in vitro* studies, calcium exhibits a 20-fold higher efficacy than phosphate in inhibiting enamel dissolution [31, 32]. Consequently, variations in calcium concentrations exert a more pronounced effect than other minerals [31].

*In vitro* investigations reveal that calcium concentration can swiftly return to its initial level once the pH surpasses 5.5, effectively halting the demineralization process. It has been observed that, after the removal of glucose, it takes approximately 40 min for the pH to exceed the critical level and around 140 min to revert to the equilibrium value of 6.5 [30].

### 1.5 Exploring the role of calcium in dental enamel

The analysis of enamel's macro-elemental composition reveals that it possesses the highest concentration of Ca2+ among all bioapatites, constituting approximately 37% of its mineral content by weight. Following closely behind, PO43- accounts for roughly 17% of the composition.

According to the literature, it has been suggested that the uptake of Ca2+ in ameloblasts is a passive process, facilitated by the extracellular to intracellular [Ca2+] gradient, with the cytosol having the lowest concentration of calcium. Subsequently, Ca2+ can be eliminated from the cytoplasm through the plasma membrane Ca2 + -ATPase (PMCA).

In a comparison of enamel's calcium concentration with those of other tissues, it becomes evident that enamel contains over nine times more Ca2+ than muscle or liver. This substantial calcium presence in enamel, approximately 90% of it, is incorporated during the maturation process, and its entry into enamel cells is of a passive nature.

Transcellular Ca2+ transport emerges as a crucial process during amelogenesis. In this process, calcium enters polarized ameloblasts at the level of the blood supply and is subsequently released into the extracellular space of enamel, where it contributes to the formation of calcium hydroxyapatite.

Hypocalcemia has a significant impact on enamel cells, resulting in the formation of cysts within the ameloblast layer and the abnormal distribution of enamel proteins [33]. Researchers have observed that low dietary Ca2+ intake in nursing mothers is the cause of hypocalcemia [34], which, in turn, leads to undermineralization of enamel in their offspring.

Fortunately, this condition was successfully addressed through a 10-day calcium supplement administered to the mothers [34]. As a result of this research, the potential existence of a stock-operated Ca2+ entry system (SOCE) was acknowledged [35]. In this proposed system, calcium enters enamel cells and is subsequently transported to the endoplasmic reticulum (ER), followed by exocytosis to the apical pole, a phenomenon known as the "transcytosis hypothesis" [17, 35].

### 1.6 Risk factors for enamel health

Dental caries is regarded as a disease resulting from the simultaneous interplay of dietary sugars, inadequate oral hygiene, and the passage of time [31]. Bacteria present in dental plaque produce organic acids, causing a drop in the pH within the plaque, a process primarily driven by the metabolism of dietary carbohydrates [31].

When the pH within the plaque repeatedly falls below the "critical pH," the enamel of the teeth initiates a process of demineralization, leading to the formation of an initial carious lesion [36]. This initial demineralization lesion is characterized by the loss of minerals from the subsurface enamel while maintaining a relatively intact surface layer [36].

Numerous studies on enamel emphasize the connection between sugar and carbohydrate consumption and the occurrence of tooth decay [37]. Any fermentable carbohydrate can be metabolized by specific oral bacteria, resulting in the production of organic acids (e.g., lactic, acetic, propionic) as byproducts [38], contributing to the formation of demineralization lesions.

The quantity of sugar in one's diet plays a crucial role in assessing the risk of caries, with research findings suggesting that both the amount of sugar consumed and the frequency of sugar consumption between meals are risk factors [37].

While the acid-induced dissolution of enamel leads to structural loss and demineralization, it is worth noting that this process can be reversed over time through remineralization. This remineralization is facilitated by calcium and phosphate from saliva within the oral environment [39].

As the acid demineralization lesion continues to progress, the structural integrity of the enamel beneath the surface deteriorates, eventually resulting in the formation of a clinically detectable cavity [31]. Extensive research and discussion have been dedicated to the role of biofilm in the etiology of caries [40].

Dental plaque constitutes a biofilm comprised of billions of bacteria, the majority of which are exclusive to the oral cavity. One of the most renowned oral bacteria is *Streptococcus mutans*, which holds a prominent role as a major etiological factor in the development of carious lesions [31].

*Streptococcus mutans* excels in producing lactic acid when exposed to sugars and polysaccharides, facilitating its adhesion to enamel and the colonization of other pathogenic microorganisms [31]. Nevertheless, it's important to note that the formation of carious enamel lesions is not solely attributed to the actions of a single microorganism. Acid production within dental plaque is a collective effort involving all acid-producing oral bacteria, collectively leading to a reduction in plaque pH [28, 31].

Below the "critical pH," typically considered to be within the range of 4.5–5.5 [28], the dental surface (DS) experiences undersaturation with respect to hydroxyapatite (HA), leading to the dissolution of enamel. The pH of dental plaque is influenced by various factors, including plaque thickness, composition, location, permeability, and the concentration of fluoride, calcium, and phosphate [29].

Following the consumption of sugar and fermentable carbohydrates, the plaque's pH rapidly plummets below pH 5.5, a process that occurs within minutes [41]. Research indicates that this acidic condition can persist for up to 20 min before gradually returning to a more neutral state. As the pH rises to values around 7 or higher, DS becomes supersaturated with respect to HA. In such conditions, enamel is capable of reclaiming mineral ions in a reparative remineralization process [41].

Repetitive exposure of enamel to low pH levels, without adequate time for repair, can shift the balance toward the formation of extensive carious lesions [41]. Salivary flow plays a crucial role in the host's resistance to caries [42].

For instance, individuals with reduced or completely absent salivary flow are often susceptible to severe caries. Saliva serves as a protective buffer against acids, contributing significantly to the maintenance of tooth integrity [31]. Moreover, in terms of enamel remineralization, saliva provides essential ions, including fluoride. It also exhibits antibacterial and antifungal properties due to the presence of lysosomes [31].

Another contributing factor to caries is the tooth's morphology and structural defects that may facilitate the accumulation of dental plaque. These factors are further influenced by the individual's behavior in terms of oral hygiene practices and regular visits to the dentist [43].

With recurrent acid attacks on enamel, the consequence is the development of porosity within the enamel structure. If these porosities are not followed by a process of remineralization and improved oral hygiene practices, they can eventually merge, leading to the formation of carious cavities [44].

For an accurate diagnosis and treatment plan, it is essential for the dentist to determine whether a lesion is active, progressing rapidly, or has ceased its development. If the lesion is confined to the enamel layer, it can be halted and may even undergo a remineralization process [45].

In Europe, the initial demineralization lesion has been referred to as the "white spot" for several years. This lesion is described as a smooth, white, or opaque area without cavities, making it prone to plaque accumulation [45].

During this white spot stage, it is possible to arrest the progression of the lesion and eliminate the porosities. If dietary chromogens become trapped during the remineralization process, it can result in the appearance of a "brown stain" [31].

Although caries can develop on any surface of the tooth, nearly 90% of cases occur on the occlusal surfaces. Research conducted over time has shown that these areas do not respond as efficiently to remineralization compared to the smooth interdental or buccal surfaces [31].

## 2. Managing dental caries

Traditional patient assessment lacks a comprehensive form that tailors prevention and treatment methods to the individual patient's caries risk. Instead, it heavily relies on invasive treatments [46].

Accurate caries risk assessment (CRA) and personalized patient management are essential for proper treatment. This approach involves a thorough analysis and control of risk factors, along with the development of customized treatment plans [46].

Several standards for classifying and managing caries currently exist. These systems were initially introduced in 2002, notably leading to the establishment of the International Caries Detection and Assessment System (ICDAS). In 2009, ICDAS underwent modifications with the addition of activity tests proposed by the International Caries Classification and Management System (ICCMS) [47]. Other systems for caries risk assessment include those by the American Dental Association (ADA), Caries Management by Risk Assessment (CAMBRA), and Cariogram [48]. Among these, the CAMBRA system stands out for its comprehensive coverage of caries risk factors [48].

### 2.1 Factors influencing caries risk

To ensure effective management of carious lesions and the selection of appropriate dental treatments, a comprehensive evaluation of the risk of dental caries is imperative. This assessment significantly influences the likelihood of future lesions and shapes the treatment plan [49]. To ascertain the accuracy of the prognosis and the impact of the chosen therapy, it is essential to reevaluate the post-treatment risk [48]. This step is a crucial component of enamel lesion management [48].

Among the various systems discussed in the previous section, the CAMBRA system stands out as the most extensive in terms of the number of risk factors associated with enamel damage, followed by ADA, Caries Risk Assessment Tool (CAT), and Cariogram [50]. Studies have indicated that the CAT and CAMBRA systems perform well for the 3-year-old age group but may not optimally predict enamel lesion prognosis [51]. Such an incomplete analysis could lead to an overestimation of caries risk in younger age groups, potentially resulting in unnecessary treatments [49].

The CAMBRA protocol is regarded as the most detailed and comprehensive approach. Within this protocol, a patient's profile is meticulously examined by evaluating risk factors such as acidogenic bacteria, fermentable carbohydrates, and low salivary flow, as well as protective factors like fluoride and antibacterial therapies [46]. Following this thorough analysis, the patient is categorized into a specific caries risk level. Based on this framework, a personalized treatment plan is devised, which may include restorative treatments, preventive therapy, or a combination of both. Treatment options may involve fluoride application, a chlorhexidine mouthwash, dental sealants, and salivary enhancers [46].

The protocol equips practitioners with all the necessary instruments for its implementation, including a questionnaire designed to identify risk factors, risk indicators, and protective factors [46]. Naturally, when employing any protocol, all patient data are taken into consideration.

Within the CAMBRA system, risk factors for enamel damage are categorized as follows:

a. CRA – the probability of the patient developing new carious lesions.

b. Preventive factors – encompassing health education and preventive therapy that aid in lesion prevention or remineralization.

c. Risk factors – factors linked to the patient's dietary and nutritional choices contributing to lesion development.

d. Caries indicators – derived from clinical examinations.

e. Carious lesion – distinguishing between cavitated and non-cavitated lesions [52].

The control of dental caries involves the application of protective factors and the reduction of pathological risk factors [52, 53]. Managing carious lesions is most effectively undertaken through a precise assessment of caries risk (CRA) and the acquisition of comprehensive information about the patient's specific risk factors.

The development of an efficient strategy to foster healthy habits among patients must also address the modification of their behavior concerning oral hygiene and periodic oral evaluations [54]. Conducting a caries risk assessment (CRA) for each individual patient is indispensable as the foundation for caries management across all age groups [52].

### 2.2 Managing caries risk assessment for individuals aged 6 and above

For the comprehensive evaluation of caries risk assessment (CRA) in patients aged 6 and older, the CAMBRA system offers the most precise guidelines:

a. Thoroughly examine the patient's dental and medical history.

b. Assess preventive measures and interventions.

c. Conduct a clinical examination to detect early enamel lesions and prevent their progression.

d. Categorize the caries risk into levels: low, moderate, high, or extreme.

e. Develop an individualized treatment plan that includes preventive or restorative measures, based on the caries risk classification in point f.

f. Implement chemical therapies, such as fluoride or other relevant substances, tailored to the detected risk factors.

g. Apply minimally invasive enamel procedures to deter enamel degradation.

h. Schedule periodic reassessments.

i. Modify the treatment plan as needed after the reassessment [52].

*2.2.1 Enhancing protective factors*

Protective factors encompass environmental, biological, or chemical elements that play a role in preventing enamel damage or facilitating its remineralization [55].

One of the most influential biological factors affecting caries risk assessment (CRA) is the patient's living environment, which includes factors such as the fluoridation of the water supply in their region or their engagement in activities like travel, work, or education in areas with similar conditions [56]. This consideration is of paramount importance because residing in such areas or using fluoride toothpaste in combination with fluoride-based mouthwash, or recently receiving topical fluoride applications, can result in an excessive influx of fluoride into the body. This excess has the potential to transform a protective factor into a potentially harmful, toxic element [56].

Regarding chemical preventive measures, the regular use of a 0.12% chlorhexidine (CHX)-based mouthwash proves beneficial on a monthly basis. Caution is warranted in this regard since overconsumption of CHX can lead to unsightly brown stains on the enamel surface [55]. The selection of treatment is contingent upon the patient's CRA level and, notably, their age [55].

*2.2.2 Factors posing risk*

The foremost risk factors include:

a. Daily consumption of carbohydrates, particularly snacks.

b. General health conditions necessitating medications that induce hyposalivation.

c. Substance abuse.

d. Inadequate oral hygiene practices.

e. Confirmed salivary dysfunction or hyposalivation.

f. Significant occlusal irregularities.

g. Extensive gingival recession with dental root exposure.

h. Use of dental appliances [1].

*2.2.3 Indicators of disease*

The dentist should clinically monitor various factors, including whether carious lesions have penetrated into the dentin, whether there are incipient demineralization lesions on intact enamel surfaces, and whether new patients within the system have received dental fillings in the past year [52].

Employing a caries risk assessment (CRA) framework facilitates the identification and categorization of patients into specific risk groups. This simplifies the dentist's oversight of the treatment protocol and the development of an effective risk factor management plan to prevent carious lesions. Additionally, it empowers the patient to gain insight into adjusting their lifestyle, especially concerning diet, nutrition, and oral hygiene, thereby influencing the progression of these lesions [52].

## 3. Utilizing nanotechnology for enhancing mineralization in dental tissues

The utilization of nanotechnology within the field of dentistry has unveiled a wealth of potential, giving rise to a novel area of research. Nanotechnology's versatile applications in dentistry encompass preventing biofilm formation, regulating the demineralization-remineralization equilibrium, combating caries [57], aiding in caries treatment, and even fabricating materials for dental implants [1].

To achieve these outcomes, calcium phosphate nanoparticles have been harnessed, displaying their ability to impede demineralization and enhance remineralization through the controlled release of calcium and phosphate ions [57].

Nanomaterials play a pivotal role in diminishing biofilm buildup, inhibiting the demineralization process, and can also be employed to counter cariogenic bacteria [1]. Substances like silver nanoparticles (Nag) and quaternary ammonium methacrylate (QAM) exhibit robust antimicrobial properties and exceptional durability, making their integration into dental materials exceptionally advantageous for enhancing antibacterial capabilities and promoting enamel remineralization [57].

Research has explored nanoparticles derived from highly soluble calcium phosphate phases, including monocalcium phosphate monohydrate, dicalcium phosphates, or amorphous calcium phosphates (ACPs), which facilitate the release of calcium and phosphate in carious lesions to promote remineralization [1, 57].

Furthermore, studies have revealed that a combination of glycine-guided hydroxyapatite and amorphous calcium phosphate (ACP) nanoparticles effectively remineralizes enamel [1, 57].

### 3.1 Biomimetic enamel mineralization

Biomineralization is a complex process that enables living organisms to accumulate inorganic ions through the involvement of protein molecules. Understanding this intricate process is vital, as it provides valuable insights into the formation of hard tissues, including bones and teeth [57].

The concept of biomimetic mineralization, which emulates the natural mineralization mechanisms of teeth, holds promise as an excellent alternative for restorative therapies when comprehended and applied [58]. Dental caries, a prevalent oral cavity ailment worldwide, arises from an imbalance between the remineralization and demineralization phases of dental hard tissue [58, 59].

Numerous remineralization approaches, such as fluoride, surfactants, electrolyte deposition, hydrothermal methods, and hydrogen peroxide, have been introduced to address initial enamel caries restoration and inhibit further demineralization [58, 59].

Tooth biomineralization encompasses both enamel and dentin mineralization. Dentin mineralization closely resembles bone mineralization, as both rely on collagen-based mineralization. In contrast, enamel lacks collagen, with amelogenin playing a pivotal role in mineralization [1].

Enamel, being an acellular tissue, presents a significant challenge for self-regeneration. Currently, the control of hydroxyapatite (HA) assembly, the fundamental component of enamel, remains undiscovered [50]. Consequently, numerous recent studies aim at biomimetic mineralization to replicate the enamel growth process [60].

To date, various typical methods for biomimetic remineralization have emerged, including ACP-induced mineralization, ion flow-induced mineralization, protein-induced mineralization, and *in situ* mineralization [60].

## 4. Conventional and contemporary approaches to preventing and assessing enamel quality decline

### 4.1 Traditional approaches to enamel examination

#### *4.1.1 Initial evaluation*

The primary objective of the examination is to visually identify alterations in enamel color and translucency, as well as changes in the enamel structure. An initial, tooth-by-tooth inspection on wet surfaces can reveal the presence of cavities, white or brown spots, and also allow for an assessment of caries activity. It is crucial, at this stage, to inspect for bacterial accumulation and signs of periodontal pathology at suspected sites.

The role of hygiene in ensuring diagnostic accuracy cannot be overstated, encompassing both direct visual assessment and the use of supplementary diagnostic methods. Utilizing magnifying loupes significantly enhances the initial detection rate of carious lesions.

Changes in color and translucency provide valuable insights into the demineralization status of the surface and subsurface areas, especially when compared to adjacent healthy regions [61].

#### *4.1.2 Radiographic evaluation*

Bitewing radiographs are the preferred technique for the early identification of carious lesions, particularly on proximal surfaces. When compared to a simple visual examination, radiographic assessments typically uncover approximately twice as many proximal lesions that extend into the dentin. Radiographs also provide the ability to estimate the depth of these carious lesions.

For the permanent dentition, it is advisable to utilize two bitewing radiographs, allowing for direct and tangential coverage of all proximal surfaces within the molar-premolar segment. It is essential to note, however, that radiography cannot detect demineralization lesions.

### 4.2 Contemporary approaches to enamel examination

#### *4.2.1 Digital scanned images*

Traditional intraoral cameras offer the capability for immediate image viewing and digital image storage. While these images are valuable for patient education on oral hygiene, they often lack the necessary quality for accurate diagnosis of carious lesions.

Chemiluminescent intraoral scanners, on the other hand, provide precise measurements of mineral loss in hard tooth structure. They rely on the absorption of fluorescent chemicals released by microorganisms in carious lesions on tooth enamel when illuminated by a diode laser with varying wavelengths [62].

In contrast, an intraoral photoluminescence camera emits visible blue light at different wavelengths to capture and encode images of teeth that exhibit fluorescence [63]. Notably, red porphyrin emits fluorescence during the early stages of carious lesions. The quantitative light-induced fluorescence method (QLF) stimulates yellow luminescence in a wavelength range above 520 nm using a 405-nm wavelength light source. The potential for early diagnosis hinges on the intensity of a tooth's natural fluorescence, which is influenced by the presence of carious lesions [64].

Optical coherence tomography (OCT) represents an even more non-invasive imaging technique with enhanced accuracy and resolution. This method is employed across various medical fields, including optometry, dental services, dermatology, and internal medicine [65].

Optical coherence tomography, in particular, stands out for its ability to detect incredibly small demineralized areas on both the surface and within the enamel, mitigating the limitations associated with other optical methods used in assessing tooth decay [66].

Extensive research in dental practice has solidified OCT's capability to produce clear images of dental tissue, offering a promising avenue for the precise measurement of early enamel carious lesions [67].

The analysis using OCT reveals mineral loss and accurately gauges the extent of demineralization within the lesion. It also allows for a more objective and precise assessment of the intensity of initial enamel carious lesions, as the quantifiable index obtained through OCT correlates significantly with enamel demineralization [65].

Additionally, various techniques, such as atomic force microscopy (AFM), microradiography, scanning electron microscopy (SEM), surface profilometry, and CLMS [61], can be employed to quantify micromorphological changes in dental enamel resulting from erosion or abrasion [61].

For over three decades, confocal laser scanning microscopy (CLSM) has been a valuable tool in dentistry, facilitating the analysis of dental materials, their properties, dental enamel, including erosion and demineralization, and even enabling the three-dimensional (3D) examination of dental plaque formation and accumulation. Furthermore, CLSM plays a vital role in the evaluation of dental implants, which have seen a surge in popularity in recent years [2].

Continuing to demonstrate its significance in dentistry, CLSM provides 3D visualizations of tooth structure, tooth surfaces, materials, and the colonization of bacteria, aiding in the exploration of tooth enamel and beyond [2].

The confocal microscope is employed to acquire high-resolution optical images, completely eliminating interference from other light wavelengths within the section. The digital nature of confocal microscope images allows for extensive post-processing and a remarkable enhancement in resolution compared to conventional microscopes [2].

In this process, the primary light source emits a point-like beam that is reflected by mirrors. Simultaneously, fluorescence, with its longer wavelength, passes through the objective lens and is captured. The fluorescence is then directed to the photodetector through the confocal objective, while fluorescence from other planes within the specimen is effectively blocked [2].

One of the standout features of CLSM is its ability to eliminate extraneous data outside the focal plane, resulting in exceptional 3D imaging performance. Unlike conventional microscopes, CLSM experiences few limitations in terms of imaging, with the main restrictions being associated with magnification and the diameter of the focusing objective [2].

Confocal laser scanning microscopy (CLSM) produces a focused beam while effectively filtering out unrelated light, allowing it to penetrate deep into the dental tissue under examination, resulting in the creation of high-quality 3D images. Both the illumination and detection are precisely directed to the same focal point, which is systematically moved across the sample's surface to collect the image data [68].

For in-depth tissue analysis in medical research, CLSM proves indispensable as it meets the specific requirements. However, it's worth noting that, to perform this analysis effectively, the sample thickness must surpass the axial resolution of the objective lens [68].

### 4.3 Conventional approaches to enamel demineralization prevention

#### *4.3.1 Fluoridation: enhancing dental health*

The outermost enamel layer can exhibit fluoride concentrations exceeding 1000 ppm, while the underlying layer typically ranges from 20 to 100 ppm (81). Nevertheless, even these concentrations fail to significantly reduce the acid solubility of artificial carbonate apatite [15].

Fluoride has been recognized as a potent agent for preventing dental caries, and the most prevalent method of prevention involves daily brushing with fluoridated toothpaste. Nonetheless, concerns arise with fluoride applications, particularly regarding potential toxicity at high doses [69].

Widespread fluoride availability has led to the emergence of fluoride-resistant strains of *S. mutans* and other oral bacterial species, diminishing the efficacy of fluoride in acid production [69].

Fluoride levels within dental biofilm and saliva have the potential to aid in enamel remineralization and inhibit demineralization [70]. Fluoride is released when the flow rate is low due to acid formation, and it can either facilitate tooth structure remineralization or impact microbial activity [70].

Professional fluoride varnish treatments have also proven effective in reducing the risk of recurrent dental caries, provided they are administered correctly and in accordance with post-lesion risk assessments [70].

#### *4.3.2 Sealing the pits and fissures: an overview*

Pit and fissure sealing has long been employed as a preventive and management strategy for dental caries in both primary and permanent teeth. The application of pit and fissure sealants on molars and premolars has proven effective in averting occlusal surface damage [70].

In line with the recommendations of the American Academy of Pediatric Dentistry (AAPD), sealants are advised exclusively for sound occlusal surfaces on permanent molars and unaffected occlusal carious lesions [71].

Although various types of sealants are available in the market, their precise effectiveness remains challenging to ascertain due to a lack of substantial evidence [72].

The sealing material must possess antibacterial properties to hinder the proliferation of microorganisms in dental plaque and safeguard healthy tissues. Furthermore, it should exhibit the appropriate consistency to readily penetrate the grooves and fissures of molars and premolars throughout their entire depth and length [73].

According to the literature, the essential characteristics of the sealing material encompass:

- Biocompatibility.
- Ease of handling and processing.
- High penetration capability and low viscosity.
- Resistance to abrasion.
- Minimal post-polymerization shrinkage.
- Esthetic appeal [73].

Initially, dental sealants were crafted using glass-ionomer cements; however, their effectiveness diminished over time. Subsequently, resin-based sealants emerged as a more enduring and widely adopted alternative. These resin-based materials are available in various forms, including opaque, translucent, and a range of colors, catering to a diverse patient base, including children [74].

Various resin-based sealant materials gradually release fluoride, thereby enhancing their dental preventive capabilities. For improved adhesion, it is essential to etch these materials with orthophosphoric acid before applying them to the enamel surface [74].

Due to the proximity of the enamel adjacent to the sealed area during the etching process, experts advise applying a fluoride layer once the sealing procedure is completed. This additional fluoride layer contributes to the remineralization of enamel affected by the acid etching process [74].

The primary purpose of the sealant is to establish a protective barrier between the most susceptible region to caries and the oral environment. It's crucial to note that the long-term effectiveness of dental sealants in preventing caries is contingent on their retention over time [75].

In general, it is recommended to apply sealants to the pits and fissures of primary molars at ages 3–4, first permanent molars at ages 6–8, and the remaining two permanent molars and premolars at ages 10–12.

A number of dentists have ceased the use of dental sealants as a treatment method, likely due to a lack of awareness concerning their effectiveness and a limited understanding of the criteria for sealant application. The proficiency and expertise in executing this medical procedure are pivotal, making the difference between a successful sealing procedure and an ineffective one [76].

For long-term effectiveness, strict adherence to the steps for preparing the dental sealant is imperative. The actual sealing of the tooth represents a critical stage. Proper isolation serves as the cornerstone for the success of any dental treatment, whether it involves sealing, composite filling, or endodontic procedures.

The indications for sealing pits and fissures encompass:

- Pits and fissures featuring intact enamel.
- Minimal opacities are also suitable for sealing.
- Deep and retentive pit and fissure morphology.

- Absence of clinical or radiographic evidence of caries.
- The tooth should have erupted recently, within the past 4 years,
- Availability of adequate isolation [77].

Contradictions for sealing pits and fissures include:
Large pits and fissures due to the potential for self-cleaning and clinical signs of interproximal caries.

- Radiographic evidence of caries.
- The presence of multiple restorations.
- Absence of any other preventive treatment.
- Partial tooth eruption.
- Inadequate isolation [77].

To ensure the enduring effectiveness of the sealing material, periodic evaluation is essential. During these assessments, the dentist should not only examine the tooth surface through tactile and visual means but also employ modern diagnostic devices like VistaCam or Diagnodent for precise evaluations [77].

The assessment should focus on the seal's integrity and its adaptation to the neighboring enamel. If there is material loss, the appearance of marginal staining, or marginal dehiscence, the dental sealant should be replaced [77].

The necessity for sealant application should be reviewed during routine preventive care sessions [70, 78].

The recommendations for using dental sealants as a preventive measure have been highly beneficial, as years of expert studies have demonstrated the method's effectiveness in preventing and halting the development of carious lesions. By filling the grooves and fissures with sealant material, children can better maintain the cleanliness of the occlusal surfaces of their posterior teeth, which are prone to retention loss [79].

However, as every study has concluded, the long-term effectiveness relies on biannual follow-ups and, if necessary, reapplication [79].

In general, it is recommended to seal the pits and fissures of primary molars at ages 3–4, first permanent molars at ages 6–8, and the remaining two permanent molars and premolars at ages 10–12.

The need for sealant application should be periodically reassessed during routine preventive care sessions [70, 78].

## 4.4 Contemporary approaches to preventing enamel demineralization

### *4.4.1 Infiltration with low-resin viscosity*

Icon, developed by DMG-Hamburg, represents a groundbreaking dental material characterized by its low viscosity. This innovative resin is ideally suited for the micro-invasive treatment of white spot lesions, demineralization, and incipient carious lesions, encompassing occlusal, buccal, and interproximal surfaces [77].

Low-resin viscosity therapy occupies an intermediate position between preventive and restorative treatments [80]. By infiltrating these lesions with resin, which acts to occlude the enamel porosities that serve as conduits for acids and minerals, caries progression can be halted [80].

Furthermore, low-viscosity infiltrating resin can also be employed to address the appearance of white spot lesions that arise post-orthodontic treatment. Research has shown that this material boasts long-term durability and produces stunning esthetic outcomes. The opacity of white spot lesions diminishes almost instantly during treatment, restoring the enamel to its natural appearance [81].

In contrast to methods such as fluoride therapy or calcium casein pastes, resin-filled microporosities do not evaporate, delivering immediate esthetic enhancements [80, 82].

In cases involving early carious lesions that are beyond the scope of fluoride therapy, resin infiltration has demonstrated its effectiveness in inhibiting the progression of caries [80, 82].

#### *4.4.2 Laser technology as a preventive approach*

Numerous *in vitro* and preliminary *in vivo* experiments have revealed the protective potential of argon laser therapy against the onset and progression of enamel carious lesions [83].

The utilization of laser technology in dental medicine represents a revolutionary approach with a wide range of applications. It not only facilitates early carious lesion detection but also offers treatment options. Additionally, oral surgery and periodontology can benefit significantly from laser technology [83].

In the realm of pediatric dentistry, laser technology holds particular appeal due to its ability to provide a relaxed, non-invasive experience for children. Moreover, it proves valuable in pediatric endodontic procedures, such as pulpotomies and pulp hemostasis [83].

Combining argon laser irradiation with topical acidulated phosphate fluoride treatment results in the creation of a protective barrier against carious lesions and a significant reduction in lesion depth [84]. This laser effectively enhances the resistance of both sound enamel and demineralized lesions to caries [83].

The laser prevents the formation of a smear layer, thereby enhancing the adhesive strength of composites. Additionally, it can be employed for laser enameloplasty before sealant placement, further bolstering caries resistance and potentially eliminating the need for traditional etching [83].

The laser also strengthens the bond between resin-based materials and the enamel surface. Using a laser before applying sealing materials proves highly advantageous, as it may obviate the need for enamel etching [83].

#### *4.4.3 Utilizing ozone therapy (O3T)*

Ozone (O3) is a highly reactive compound consisting of three oxygen atoms, acting as both an oxidant and oxidizer [85]. Ozone therapy, as a non-invasive alternative for addressing tooth decay, offers distinctive advantages when compared to other available treatments. The primary objective of ozone therapy for carious lesions is to diminish the causative microbiota, reduce risk factors, arrest the caries process, and promote remineralization. Enamel remains vulnerable throughout one's life, continually exposed to the oral environment. The acidic conditions created by bacteria, dietary factors, and beverages contribute to dental issues, affecting four out of five primary teeth in children and over half of permanent teeth in adults [11, 86]. Given that enamel is categorized as acellular tissue, it lacks the capacity for self-regeneration or reshaping, making the lesions irreversible and necessitating restoration with artificial materials.

A key challenge in non-invasive approaches to prevent carious lesions and promote enamel remineralization lies in controlling dental plaque. Ozone can remove proteins from carious lesions, facilitating the diffusion of calcium and phosphate ions through the lesions, thereby promoting remineralization [87]. Moreover, ozone offers environmental benefits, as it rapidly degrades and exhibits low cytotoxicity when in contact with organic compounds. These characteristics suggest a promising future for ozone in restorative and preventive dentistry [87].

Due to its potent oxidation capabilities, ozone can oxidize bacterial cell walls, leading to lysis, and can transform the pyruvic acid produced by bacteria into acetic acid and carbon dioxide, thereby halting or reversing the progression of caries. While the antimicrobial properties of ozone are well documented [85, 88–91], its potential for remineralization by enhancing dentin tubule permeability is less explored. As a demineralizing agent, ozone appears to enhance the diffusion of salivary ions to the degraded dentin surface, facilitating remineralization [85, 92–94]. In this context, ozone can counteract the acidic proteins produced by cariogenic bacteria, which are responsible for osmotic stimulation, leading to fluid movement within dentin tubules and resulting in hypersensitivity [93–95].

Considering the various therapeutic effects of ozone outlined above, it is important to note that these effects arise from diverse mechanisms of action, including:

- Antimicrobial properties: Ozone acts as an antimicrobial agent by destroying viral capsids and disrupting the reproductive cycle through peroxidation.

- Immune modulation and antioxidant activity: Ozone serves as an immune modulator and antioxidant agent by stimulating immunoglobulin synthesis, maintaining cell redox balance, and increasing cellular levels of glutathione (GSH) peroxidase.

- Anti-hypoxic effect: Ozone enhances oxygen saturation in hemoglobin, thereby counteracting hypoxia.

- Anti-inflammatory action: Ozone's anti-inflammatory impact is achieved by influencing the synthesis of interleukins, prostaglandins, and leukotrienes.

- Bioenergetics enhancement: Ozone activates protein synthesis and boosts cellular metabolism, contributing to its bioenergetic effect.

- Detoxification: Ozone promotes cellular aerobic processes, including the Krebs cycle, glycolysis, and fatty acid oxidation, thus facilitating detoxification.

- Biosynthetic function: Ozone enhances the metabolism of carbohydrates, proteins, and lipids, impacting biosynthetic processes [96].

Ozone can be applied to the tooth's surface using either gas or water delivery methods. It possesses robust bio-oxidative properties, is highly bactericidal, and has found utility in dentistry for the treatment of dental caries in both enamel and dentin, as well as for addressing root caries and dental hypersensitivity [92].

## 5. Conclusions

In conclusion, the current era, marked by rapid technological advancements, has paradoxically witnessed a concerning surge in dental injuries across all age groups. The persistence of such issues prompts a critical evaluation of our existing treatment methodologies and problem-solving approaches. While carious lesions are officially recognized as a preventable disease, the ongoing escalation of dental problems necessitates a reexamination of preventive strategies. Fluoridation, sealing techniques, and maintenance of oral hygiene are conventional methods that have endured the test of time. However, the evolving landscape introduces innovative approaches like biomimetic enamel mineralization, offering promising alternatives for restorative therapies. The integration of digital scanned images, chemiluminescent intraoral scanners, intraoral photoluminescence cameras, and optical coherence tomography in enamel examination represents a significant stride toward non-invasive and accurate diagnostics. The multifaceted nature of enamel demineralization prevention requires a holistic approach, encompassing dietary adjustments, individual risk factor management, and education to induce transformative changes in patient behavior. In this ever-evolving landscape, the identification and regulation of individual-level risk factors, coupled with advancements in biomimetic mineralization and cutting-edge diagnostic technologies, pave the way for a comprehensive and effective paradigm in the prevention and management of enamel demineralization.

## Conflict of interest

The authors declare no conflict of interest.

## Author details

Atena Galuscan[1,2], Daniela Jumanca[1,2] and Ramona Dumitrescu[1,2*]

1 Department of Preventive, Community Dentistry and Oral Health, Department I, University of Medicine and Pharmacy "Victor Babes", Timisoara, Romania

2 Translational and Experimental Clinical Research Centre in Oral Health, Department of Preventive, Community Dentistry and Oral Health, University of Medicine and Pharmacy "Victor Babes", Timisoara, Romania

*Address all correspondence to: dumitrescu.ramona@umft.ro

## References

[1] Sharma V, Srinivasan A, Nikolajeff F, Kumar S. Biomineralization process in hard tissues: The interaction complexity within protein and inorganic counterparts. Acta Biomaterialia. 2021;**120**:20-37. DOI: 10.1016/j.actbio.2020.04.049

[2] Chen H, Tang Z, Liu J, Sun K, Chang S-R, Peters MC, et al. Acellular synthesis of a human enamel-like microstructure. Advanced Materials. 2006;**18**:1846-1851. DOI: 10.1002/adma.200502401

[3] Wang S, Zhang L, Chen W, Jin H, Zhang Y, Wu L, et al. Rapid regeneration of enamel-like-oriented inorganic crystals by using rotary evaporation. Materials Science and Engineering: C. 2020;**115**:111141. DOI: 10.1016/j.msec.2020.111141

[4] Zou Z, Liu X, Chen L, Lin K, Chang J. Dental enamel-like hydroxyapatite transformed directly from Monetite. Journal of Materials Chemistry. 2012;**22**:22637. DOI: 10.1039/c2jm35430f

[5] Zhang YY, Li QL, Wong HM. Cell-free biomimetic mineralization strategies to regenerate the enamel microstructure. Crystals. 2021;**11**:1385. DOI: 10.3390/cryst11111385

[6] Beniash E, Stifler CA, Sun C-Y, Jung GS, Qin Z, Buehler MJ, et al. The hidden structure of human enamel. Nature Communications. 2019;**10**:4383. DOI: 10.1038/s41467-019-12185-7

[7] Rivera C, Arola D, Ossa A. Indentation damage and crack repair in human enamel. Journal of the Mechanical Behavior of Biomedical Materials. 2013;**21**:178-184. DOI: 10.1016/j.jmbbm.2013.02.020

[8] Solaymani S, Ghoranneviss M, Elahi SM, Shafiekhani A, Kulesza S, Ţălu Ş, et al. The relation between structural, Rugometric and fractal characteristics of hard dental tissues at micro and Nano levels. Microscopy Research & Techniques. 2019;**82**:421-428. DOI: 10.1002/jemt.23183

[9] Yamamoto T, Hasegawa T, Yamamoto T, Hongo H, Amizuka N. Histology of human cementum: Its structure, function, and development. Japanese Dental Science Review. 2016;**52**:63-74. DOI: 10.1016/j.jdsr.2016.04.002

[10] Balhuc S, Campian R, Labunet A, Negucioiu M, Buduru S, Kui A. Dental applications of systems based on hydroxyapatite nanoparticles—An evidence-based update. Crystals. 2021;**11**:674. DOI: 10.3390/cryst11060674

[11] Lacruz RS, Habelitz S, Wright JT, Paine ML. Dental enamel formation and implications for oral health and disease. Physiological Reviews. 2017;**97**:939-993. DOI: 10.1152/physrev.00030.2016

[12] Lacruz RS, Smith CE, Bringas P, Chen Y, Smith SM, Snead ML, et al. Identification of novel candidate genes involved in mineralization of dental enamel by genome-wide transcript profiling. Journal Cellular Physiology. 2012;**227**:2264-2275. DOI: 10.1002/jcp.22965

[13] Eckstein M, Aulestia FJ, Nurbaeva MK, Lacruz RS. Altered $Ca^{2+}$ signaling in enamelopathies. Biochimica et Biophysica Acta (BBA) – Molecular Cell Research. 2018;**1865**:1778-1785. DOI: 10.1016/j.bbamcr.2018.04.013

[14] Kong Z, Lin J, Yu M, Yu L, Li J, Weng W, et al. Enhanced loading and

controlled release of rhBMP-2 in thin mineralized collagen coatings with the aid of chitosan nanospheres and its biological evaluations. Journal of Materials Chemistry B. 2014;**2**:4572-4582. DOI: 10.1039/C4TB00404C

[15] Johnsson M, Richardson CF, Bergey EJ, Levine MJ, Nancollas GH. The effects of human salivary cystatins and statherin on hydroxyapatite crystallization. Archives of Oral Biology. 1991;**36**:631-636. DOI: 10.1016/0003-9969(91)90014-L

[16] Boyde A. Microstructure of enamel. In: Chadwick DJ, Cardew G, editors. Novartis Foundation Symposia. Wiley; 2007. pp. 18-31. ISBN 978-0-471-96872-6. Available from: https://www.wiley.com/en-be/Dental+Enamel-p-9780470515303

[17] Eckstein M, Lacruz RS. CRAC channels in dental enamel cells. Cell Calcium. 2018;**75**:14-20. DOI: 10.1016/j.ceca.2018.07.012

[18] Kallenbach E. Fine structure of the stratum intermedium, stellate reticulum, and outer enamel epithelium in the enamel organ of the kitten. Journal of Anatomy. 1978;**126**:247-260

[19] Nanci A, TenCate AR. Ten Cate's Oral Histology: Development, Structure, and Function. 9th ed. St. Louis, Missouri: Elsevier; 2018. ISBN 978-0-323-48524-1

[20] Fukae M, Tanabe T, Uchida T, Yamakoshi Y, Shimizu M. Enamelins in the newly formed bovine enamel. Calcified Tissue International. 1993;**53**:257-261. DOI: 10.1007/BF01320911

[21] Bone and Joint Research Group, Centre for Human Development, Stem Cells and Regeneration, Human Development and Health, Institute of Developmental Sciences, University of Southampton Medical School, Southampton, U.K. Smith E, Kanczler J, Oreffo R. A new take on an old story: Chick limb organ culture for skeletal niche development and regenerative medicine evaluation. eCM. 2013;**26**:91-106. DOI: 10.22203/eCM.v026a07

[22] Bentmann A, Kawelke N, Moss D, Zentgraf H, Bala Y, Berger I, et al. Circulating fibronectin affects bone matrix, whereas osteoblast fibronectin modulates osteoblast function. Journal of Bone & Mineral Research. 2010;**25**:706-715. DOI: 10.1359/jbmr.091011

[23] Liao H-T, Chen C-T. Osteogenic potential: Comparison between bone marrow and adipose-derived mesenchymal stem cells. World Journal of Stem Cells. 2014;**6**:288-295. DOI: 10.4252/wjsc.v6.i3.288

[24] Krzyściak W, Jurczak A, Kościelniak D, Bystrowska B, Skalniak A. The virulence of *Streptococcus mutans* and the ability to form biofilms. European Journal of Clinical Microbiology & Infectious Diseases. 2014;**33**:499-515. DOI: 10.1007/s10096-013-1993-7

[25] Li X, Chang W-C, Chao YJ, Wang R, Chang M. Nanoscale structural and mechanical characterization of a natural nanocomposite material: The Shell of red abalone. Nano Letters. 2004;**4**:613-617. DOI: 10.1021/nl049962k

[26] Plunkett N, O'Brien FJ. Bioreactors in tissue engineering. THC. 2011;**19**:55-69. DOI: 10.3233/THC-2011-0605

[27] Yamakoshi Y, Richardson AS, Nunez SM, Yamakoshi F, Milkovich RN, Hu JC, et al. Enamel proteins and proteases in Mmp20 and Klk4 null and double-null mice. European Journal of Oral Sciences. 2011;**119**:206-216. DOI: 10.1111/j.1600-0722.2011.00866.x

[28] Dawes C. What is the critical pH and why does a tooth dissolve in acid? Journal of the Canadian Dental Association. 2003;**69**:722-724

[29] Kurtz KS. Diagnosis and risk prediction of dental caries, volume 2. Journal of Prosthodontics. 2002;**11**:321-323. DOI: 10.1111/j.1532-849X.2002.321_1.x

[30] Ilie O, Van Loosdrecht MCM, Picioreanu C. Mathematical modelling of tooth demineralisation and pH profiles in dental plaque. Journal of Theoretical Biology. 2012;**309**:159-175. DOI: 10.1016/j.jtbi.2012.05.024

[31] West NX, Joiner A. Enamel mineral loss. Journal of Dentistry. 2014;**42**:S2-S11. DOI: 10.1016/S0300-5712(14)50002-4

[32] Lynch RJM, Ten Cate JM. The anti-caries efficacy of calcium carbonate-based fluoride toothpastes. International Dental Journal. 2005;**55**:175-178. DOI: 10.1111/j.1875-595X.2005.tb00055.x

[33] Nanci A, Mocetti P, Sakamoto Y, Kunikata M, Lozupone E, Bonucci E. Morphological and immunocytochemical analyses on the effects of diet-induced hypocalcemia on enamel maturation in the rat incisor. The Journal of Histochemistry and Cytochemistry. 2000;**48**:1043-1057. DOI: 10.1177/002215540004800803

[34] Bonucci E, Lozupone E, Silvestrini G, Favia A, Mocetti P. Morphological studies of hypomineralized enamel of rat pups on calcium-deficient diet, and of its changes after return to normal diet. The Anatomical Record. 1994;**239**:379-395. DOI: 10.1002/ar.1092390405

[35] Hubbard MJ. Calcium transport across the dental enamel epithelium. Critical Reviews in Oral Biology & Medicine. 2000;**11**:437-466. DOI: 10.1177/10454411000110040401

[36] Ilie O, Van Turnhout AG, Van Loosdrecht MCM, Picioreanu C. Numerical modelling of tooth enamel subsurface lesion formation induced by dental plaque. Caries Research. 2014;**48**:73-89. DOI: 10.1159/000354123

[37] Gupta N, Singh R, Gambhir N, Chakraborty S. Efficacy of silver diamine fluoride on *Streptococcus mutans* count present in saliva. International Journal of Clinical Pediatric Dentistry. 2021;**14**:700-704. DOI: 10.5005/jp-journals-10005-2037

[38] Dawasaz AA, Togoo RA, Mahmood Z, Azlina A, Thirumulu Ponnuraj K. Effectiveness of self-assembling peptide (P11-4) in dental hard tissue conditions: A comprehensive review. Polymers. 2022;**14**:792. DOI: 10.3390/polym14040792

[39] Hemingway CA, Parker DM, Addy M, Barbour ME. Erosion of enamel by non-carbonated soft drinks with and without toothbrushing abrasion. British Dental Journal. 2006;**201**:447-450. DOI: 10.1038/sj.bdj.4814073

[40] Peterson SN, Snesrud E, Schork NJ, Bretz WA. Dental caries pathogenicity: A genomic and metagenomic perspective. International Dental Journal. 2011;**61**:11-22. DOI: 10.1111/j.1875-595X.2011.00025.x

[41] Featherstone JDB. Remineralization, the natural caries repair process—The need for new approaches. Advances in Dental Research. 2009;**21**:4-7. DOI: 10.1177/0895937409335590

[42] Stookey GK. The effect of saliva on dental caries. The Journal of the American Dental Association. 2008;**139**:11S-17S. DOI: 10.14219/jada.archive.2008.0347

[43] Duggal MS, Nikolopoulou A, Tahmassebi JF. The additional effect of ozone in combination with adjunct remineralisation products on inhibition of demineralisation of the dental hard tissues in situ. Journal of Dentistry. 2012;**40**:934-940. DOI: 10.1016/j.jdent.2012.07.012

[44] Banerjee A. Minimal intervention dentistry: Part 7. Minimally invasive operative caries management: Rationale and techniques. British Dental Journal. 2013;**214**:107-111. DOI: 10.1038/sj.bdj.2013.106

[45] Mohamed AM, Wong KH, Lee WJ, Marizan Nor M, Mohd Hussaini H, Rosli TI. *In vitro* study of white spot lesion: Maxilla and mandibular teeth. The Saudi Dental Journal. 2018;**30**:142-150. DOI: 10.1016/j.sdentj.2017.12.001

[46] Coelho A, Amaro I, Iunes T, Paula A, Marto CM, Saraiva J, et al. CAMBRA Protocol Efficacy: A Systematic Review and Critical Appraisal. Journal of Dentistry (Basel). 2022;**10**(6):97. DOI: 10.3390/dj10060097. PMID: 35735639; PMCID: PMC9221725

[47] Cheng J, Chaffee BW, Cheng NF, Gansky SA, Featherstone JDB. Understanding treatment effect mechanisms of the CAMBRA randomized trial in reducing caries increment. Journal of Dental Research. 2015;**94**:44-51. DOI: 10.1177/0022034514555365

[48] Featherstone JDB, Domejean-Orliaguet S, Jenson L, Wolff M, Young DA. Caries risk assessment in practice for age 6 through adult. Journal of the California Dental Association. 2007;**35**(703-707):710-713

[49] Cheng L, Zhang L, Yue L, Ling J, Fan M, Yang D, et al. Expert consensus on dental caries management. International Journal of Oral Science. 2022;**14**:17. DOI: 10.1038/s41368-022-00167-3

[50] Tellez M, Gomez J, Pretty I, Ellwood R, Ismail A. Evidence on existing caries risk assessment systems: Are they predictive of future caries? Community Dentistry and Oral Epidemiology. 2013;**41**:67-78. DOI: 10.1111/cdoe.12003

[51] Gao X, Di Wu I, Lo ECM, Chu CH, Hsu CS, Wong MCM. Validity of caries risk assessment programmes in preschool children. Journal of Dentistry. 2013;**41**:787-795. DOI: 10.1016/j.jdent.2013.06.005

[52] Featherstone JDB, Crystal YO, Alston P, Chaffee BW, Doméjean S, Rechmann P, et al. Evidence-based caries management for all ages-practical guidelines. Frontiers in Oral Health. 2021;**2**:657518. DOI: 10.3389/froh.2021.657518

[53] Rechmann P, Chaffee BW, Rechmann BMT, Featherstone JDB. Changes in carries risk in a practice-based randomized controlled trial. Advances in Dental Research. 2018;**29**:15-23. DOI: 10.1177/0022034517737022

[54] Okunseri C, Gonzalez C, Hodgson B. Children's oral health assessment, prevention, and treatment. Pediatric Clinics of North America. 2015;**62**:1215-1226. DOI: 10.1016/j.pcl.2015.05.010

[55] Featherstone JDB, White JM, Hoover CI, Rapozo-Hilo M, Weintraub JA, Wilson RS, et al. A randomized clinical trial of anticaries therapies targeted according to risk assessment (caries management by risk assessment). Caries Research. 2012;**46**:118-129. DOI: 10.1159/000337241

[56] Curnow MMT, Pine CM, Burnside G, Nicholson JA, Chesters RK, Huntington E. A randomised controlled trial of the efficacy of supervised

toothbrushing in high-caries-risk children. Caries Research. 2002;**36**:294-300. DOI: 10.1159/000063925

[57] Cheng L, Zhang K, Weir MD, Melo MAS, Zhou X, Xu HH. Nanotechnology strategies for antibacterial and remineralizing composites and adhesives to tackle dental caries. Nanomedicine. 2015;**10**:627-641. DOI: 10.2217/nnm.14.191

[58] Zafar MS, Amin F, Fareed MA, Ghabbani H, Riaz S, Khurshid Z, et al. Biomimetic aspects of restorative dentistry biomaterials. Biomimetics. 2020;**5**:34. DOI: 10.3390/biomimetics5030034

[59] Wang J, Liu Q, Guo Z, Pan H, Liu Z, Tang R. Progress on biomimetic mineralization and materials for hard tissue regeneration. ACS Biomaterials Science & Engineering. 2023;**9**:1757-1773. DOI: 10.1021/acsbiomaterials.1c01070

[60] Zhao H, Liu S, Lu J, Yang X, Yang Z, Li F, et al. Natural tooth enamel and its analogs. Cell Reports Physical Science. 2022;**3**:100945. DOI: 10.1016/j.xcrp.2022.100945

[61] Santiago, Sl PV. Methodologies to analyze the micromorphological alterations of enamel subjected to abrasion/erosion. Dentistry. 2014;**4**(9):1000255. DOI: 10.4172/2161-1122.1000255. 1000255, ISSN:2161-1122

[62] Hibst R, Paulus R, Lussi A. Detection of occlusal carries by laser fluorescence: Basic and clinical investigations. Medical Laser Application. 2001;**16**:205-213. DOI: 10.1078/1615-1615-00024

[63] Rodrigues JA, Hug I, Diniz MB, Lussi A. Performance of fluorescence methods, radiographic examination and ICDAS II on occlusal surfaces *in vitro*. Caries Research. 2008;**42**:297-304. DOI: 10.1159/000148162

[64] Thanh MTG, Van Toan N, Toan DTT, Thang NP, Dong NQ, Dung NT, et al. Diagnostic value of fluorescence methods, visual inspection and photographic visual examination in initial caries lesion: A systematic review and meta-analysis. Dentistry Journal. 2021;**9**:30. DOI: 10.3390/dj9030030

[65] Shi B, Niu J, Zhou X, Dong X. Quantitative assessment methods of early enamel caries with optical coherence tomography: A review. Applied Sciences. 2022;**12**:8780. DOI: 10.3390/app12178780

[66] Yang Z, Shang J, Liu C, Zhang J, Hou F, Liang Y. Intraoperative imaging of oral-maxillofacial lesions using optical coherence tomography. Journal of Innovative Optical Health Sciences. 2020;**13**:2050010. DOI: 10.1142/S1793545820500108

[67] Shimada Y, Sadr A, Burrow MF, Tagami J, Ozawa N, Sumi Y. Validation of swept-source optical coherence tomography (SS-OCT) for the diagnosis of occlusal caries. Journal of Dentistry. 2010;**38**:655-665. DOI: 10.1016/j.jdent.2010.05.004

[68] Chen Z, Miao Z, Zhang P, Xiao H, Liu H, Ding C, et al. Bioinspired enamel-like oriented minerals on general surfaces: Towards improved mechanical properties. Journal of Materials Chemistry B. 2019;**7**:5237-5244. DOI: 10.1039/C9TB00676A

[69] Bijle MNA, Ekambaram M, Lo EC, Yiu CKY. The combined enamel remineralization potential of arginine and fluoride toothpaste. Journal of Dentistry. 2018;**76**:75-82. DOI: 10.1016/j.jdent.2018.06.009

[70] Zou J, Du Q, Ge L, Wang J, Wang X, Li Y, et al. Expert consensus on early childhood caries management. International Journal of Oral

Science. 2022;**14**:35. DOI: 10.1038/s41368-022-00186-0

[71] Wright JT, Crall JJ, Fontana M, Gillette EJ, Nový BB, Dhar V, et al. Evidence-based clinical practice guideline for the use of pit-and-fissure sealants. The Journal of the American Dental Association. 2016;**147**:672-682.e12. DOI: 10.1016/j.adaj.2016.06.001

[72] Ahovuo-Saloranta A, Forss H, Walsh T, Nordblad A, Mäkelä M, Worthington HV. Pit and fissure sealants for preventing dental decay in permanent teeth. Cochrane Database of Systematic Reviews. 2017;**7**:CD001830. DOI: 10.1002/14651858.CD001830.pub5

[73] Elliott AD. Confocal microscopy: Principles and modern practices. CP Cytometry. 2020;**92**:e68. DOI: 10.1002/cpcy.68

[74] Naaman R, El-Housseiny A, Alamoudi N. The use of pit and fissure sealants—A literature review. Dentistry Journal. 2017;**5**:34. DOI: 10.3390/dj5040034

[75] Condò R, Cioffi A, Riccio A, Totino M, Condò SG, Cerroni L. Sealants in dentistry: A systematic review of the literature. Oral & Implantology (Rome). 2013;**6**:67-74

[76] Canga M, Malagnino VA, Malagnino I, Malagnino G. Effectiveness of sealants treatment in permanent molars: A longitudinal study. International Journal of Clinical Pediatric Dentistry. 2021;**14**:41-45. DOI: 10.5005/jp-journals-10005-1878

[77] Marya C, Bhatia HP, Gupta P, Dhingra S, Kataria S, Lnu M. Pit and fissure sealants: An unused caries prevention tool. Journal of Oral Health and Community Dentistry. 2010;**4**:1-6. DOI: 10.5005/johcd-4-1-1

[78] Sasa I, Donly KJ. Sealants: A review of the materials and utilization. Journal of the California Dental Association. 2010;**38**:730-734

[79] Cvikl B, Moritz A, Bekes K. Pit and fissure sealants—A comprehensive review. Dentistry Journal. 2018;**6**:18. DOI: 10.3390/dj6020018

[80] Mandava J. Microhardness and penetration of artificial white spot lesions treated with resin or colloidal silica infiltration. JCDR. 2017;**11**(4):ZC142-ZC146. DOI: 10.7860/JCDR/2017/25512.9706

[81] Kannan A, Padmanabhan S. Comparative evaluation of icon® resin infiltration and Clinpro™ XT varnish on colour and fluorescence changes of white spot lesions: A randomized controlled trial. Progress in Orthodontics. 2019;**20**:23. DOI: 10.1186/s40510-019-0276-y

[82] Kielbassa AM, Muller J, Gernhardt CR. Closing the gap between oral hygiene and minimally invasive dentistry: A review on the resin infiltration technique of incipient (proximal) enamel lesions. Quintessence International. 2009;**40**:663-681

[83] Prathima GS, Bhadrashetty D, Babu SBU, Disha P. Microdentistry with lasers. Journal of International Oral Health. 2015;**7**:134-137

[84] Westerman GH, Hicks MJ, Flaitz CM, Ellis RW, Powell GL. Argon laser irradiation and fluoride treatment effects on caries-like enamel lesion formation in primary teeth: An *in vitro* study. American Journal of Dentistry. 2004;**17**:241-244

[85] Suh Y, Patel S, Kaitlyn R, Gandhi J, Joshi G, Smith N, et al. Clinical utility of ozone therapy in dental and oral medicine.

Medical Gas Research. 2019;**9**:163. DOI: 10.4103/2045-9912.266997

[86] Kreulen CM, Van'T Spijker A, Rodriguez JM, Bronkhorst EM, Creugers NHJ, Bartlett DW. Systematic review of the prevalence of tooth wear in children and adolescents. Caries Research. 2010;**44**:151-159. DOI: 10.1159/000308567

[87] Elsayad II. Chemical analysis and surface morphology of enamel following ozone application with different concentrations and exposure times. Journal of Advanced Research. 2011;**2**:131-136. DOI: 10.1016/j.jare.2010.10.001

[88] Viebahn-Haensler R, León Fernández OS, Ozone in Medicine. The low-dose ozone concept and its basic biochemical mechanisms of action in chronic inflammatory diseases. International Journal of Molecular Sciences. 2021;**22**:7890. DOI: 10.3390/ijms22157890

[89] Sen S, Sen S. Ozone therapy a new vista in dentistry: Integrated review. Medical Gas Research. 2020;**10**:189. DOI: 10.4103/2045-9912.304226

[90] Elvis A, Ekta J. Ozone therapy: A clinical review. Journal of Natural Science, Biology and Medicine. 2011;**2**:66. DOI: 10.4103/0976-9668.82319

[91] Santos GM, Pacheco RL, Bussadori SK, Santos EM, Riera R, Latorraca, C DOC, et al. Effectiveness and safety of ozone therapy in dental caries treatment: Systematic review and meta-analysis. Journal of Evidence Based Dental Practice. 2020;**20**:101472. DOI: 10.1016/j.jebdp.2020.101472

[92] Almaz ME, Sönmez IŞ. Ozone therapy in the management and prevention of caries. Journal of the Formosan Medical Association. 2015;**114**:3-11. DOI: 10.1016/j.jfma.2013.06.020

[93] Raafat Abdelaziz R, Mosallam RS, Yousry MM. Tubular occlusion of simulated hypersensitive dentin by the combined use of ozone and desensitizing agents. Acta Odontologica Scandinavica. 2011;**69**:395-400. DOI: 10.3109/00016357.2011.572290

[94] Lena K, Marianne K. Ozone treatment on dentin hypersensitivity surfaces – A pilot study. Todentj. 2017;**11**:65-70. DOI: 10.2174/1874210601711010065

[95] Luppieri V, Manfra A, Ronfani L, Chermetz M, Cadenaro M. Ozone therapy for early childhood caries (ECC) treatment: An *in vivo* prospective study. Applied Sciences. 1964;**2022**:12. DOI: 10.3390/app12041964

[96] Floare AD, Scurtu AD, Balean OI, Chioran D, Buzatu R, Sava Rosianu R, et al. The biological effects of ozone gas on soft and hard dental tissues and the impact on human gingival fibroblasts and gingival keratinocytes. PRO. 2021;**9**:1978. DOI: 10.3390/pr9111978

## Chapter 5

# White Spot Lesions of Carious Etiology

*Lavinia Cosmina Ardelean, Codruta Victoria Tigmeanu, Alexandra Roi and Laura-Cristina Rusu*


## Abstract

Demineralization-induced white spot lesions (WSL) are early non-cavitated carious lesions, representing the earliest stage of tooth decay, and appear as opaque, milky, porous areas, with a depth of only 40–130 μm. They are frequently found postfixed orthodontic treatment, because of the retentive nature of brackets and wires, and the inherent difficulties in maintaining proper oral hygiene, but can be found in non-orthodontic patients, as well. The main concern is of esthetic nature, but untreated WSL may evolve in dental caries, with important structural and functional consequences. The treatment approach more often uses conservative methods such as remineralization, microabrasion, tooth whitening, and resin infiltration, but, depending on the case, resin restorations and veneers may be involved. This chapter aims to discuss their etiology, characteristics and diagnosis, prevention and treatment methods, and to present three clinical cases of demineralized induced WSL, of orthodontic and non-orthodontic origin, treated by means of a microinvasive method, namely resin infiltration.


**Keywords:** white spot lesion, WSL, enamel, demineralization, remineralization, resin infiltration, microabrasion, fluoridation

## 1. Introduction

White spot lesions (WSL) are of different etiologies and can be categorized as non-carious (due to fluorosis or developmental enamel defects such as amelogenesis imperfecta and molar incisor hypomineralization) and carious (due to localized demineralization of the enamel in non-orthodontic patients and localized areas of demineralization related to orthodontic appliances). The etiology of the WSL is of utmost importance for the treatment outcome and esthetic improvement [1].

Fluorosis results from excessive fluoride intake during tooth development and may manifest as a discoloration ranging from white spots to brown staining, accompanied by pits or cracks.

Amelogenesis imperfecta is an enamel development defect, that can be classified into three types: hypomineralized, hypomaturated, and hypoplastic.

Enamel hypoplasia is due to affected matrix formation, hypomineralization is the effect of maturation disturbance, while hypomaturation is caused by the reduced mineral deposition in the late stages of mineralization. Enamel hypoplasia appears as pits, grooves, and thin or missing enamel, hypomineralization is characterized by soft enamel, and hypomaturation by altered translucency of the entire tooth [2].

Molar incisor hypomineralization is a developmental condition that involves first or second permanent molars and permanent incisors, and appears as different-colored and demarcated enamel opacities, occasionally undergoing posteruptive breakdown [3].

These developmental enamel defects not only impair the esthetics but also exert significant effects on tooth sensitivity and function, being related to the early appearance of dental caries and malocclusion [4].

WSL of carious etiology are being associated with demineralization, and described as early non-cavitated carious lesions, representing the earliest stage of tooth decay. Demineralization related to orthodontic appliances does not represent a distinct type of caries, being the result of the earliest carious process occurring around fixed orthodontic appliances.

According to Fejerskov et al. [5], demineralization-induced WSL can be defined as the "first sign of a caries lesion on enamel that can be detected with the naked eye." Their appearance, as white, chalky, and opaque spots, is due to the mineral loss that occurs in the surface and subsurface of the enamel, being, in fact, an optical phenomenon, and it is highlighted by drying. They are rough and porous compared with WSL of non-carious etiology, which are typically smooth and shiny. The prevalence of demineralized-induced WSL has increased lately, particularly in orthodontic patients. Left untreated, WSL can eventually develop into dental cavities [6].

Regardless of their etiology, white spot lesions may cause functional and esthetic concerns, strongly depending on their extent, depth, and color. Differential diagnosis, based on a thorough review of dental and medical history, and clinical evaluation of the location, form, symmetry, color, opacity, depth, and texture are essential in making a decision on the most appropriate type of treatment [1].

From a clinical point of view, in case of demineralization-induced WSL, preventive procedures, such as proper oral hygiene, non-cariogenic diet, and topical fluoride application are of utmost importance [2].

Treatment of WSL includes various methods, ranging from conservative to more invasive ones, such as composite restorations, veneers, and even crowns, which are mainly indicated in severe enamel discoloration or structural damage, which can be found more frequently in non-carious WSL. To fully mask the discoloration, a thicker composite layer is often needed, which may leave the tooth bulky. The esthetic outcome of veneers and crowns is definitely a good one, but they involve extensive dental tissue sacrifice, which is justified only in severe WSL cases, which cannot be treated by more conservative methods. Conservative treatment methods include remineralization, microabrasion, tooth whitening, and resin infiltration.

This chapter will further refer to *WSL of carious etiology (demineralization induced) only* (further referred to as WSL), aiming to discuss their etiology, characteristics and diagnosis, prevention and treatment methods, and to present three clinical cases of demineralized induced WSL, of orthodontic and non-orthodontic origin, treated by means of a microinvasive method, namely resin infiltration.

## 2. Etiology

WSL are the result of the bacterial acid attack of the dental biofilm. A poor oral hygiene, an insufficient salivary flow, which does not support self-cleansing, and a high-carb diet, combined with frequent exposure to fermentable carbohydrates, play their role in providing a favorable environment for developing and multiplying of cariogenic bacteria [7].

The most predisposed to WSL occurrence are highly retentive areas, which are difficult to clean and most predisposed to stagnating dental biofilm, such as neighboring areas to fixed orthodontic appliances. A total of 50% of orthodontic patients have one or more WSL, compared to 11% non-orthodontic ones [7].

Individuals exhibit different levels of caries risk, therefore a patient with an apparently acceptable dental hygiene may develop the same amount of enamel lesions as one with a poor dental hygiene. The salivary flow, the composition of the saliva, the enamel structure, the diet, as well as the genetic predisposal, are factors that may influence the individual response to acid attack [7].

Acidogenic bacteria, namely *Streptococcus mutans and Lactobacilli* are the primary microbial agents involved in the outbreak and development of caries. At the surface of sound enamel, the majority of the microflora is composed of non-mutans *streptococci*, the acidity being mild and of low frequency. This situation is prone to modification in case of a diet rich in fermentable carbohydrates and favors the development of an acidogenic microflora, resulting in higher levels of enamel demineralization [8, 9].

## 3. Characteristics and diagnosis

The enamel demineralization-remineralization is a dynamic, continuous, simultaneous, or alternating process. Demineralization is induced by pathological factors such as acidogenic bacteria, low salivary flow, and high-carb diet, while remineralization is due to protective factors such as antibacterial agents, sufficient salivary secretion, remineralizing ions, and specific dietary nutrients. An altered balance between demineralization and remineralization results in caries initiate or arrest [5, 7].

However, when the pH is low for a longer period of time, demineralization becomes dominant, the quantity of ions that depart the enamel surface being higher than the quantity which returns. The first demineralization stage is represented by the dissolution of the interprismatic substance. The mineral loss broadly varies between 10 and 70%. The early non-cavitated carious lesion is characterized by a depth of only 40–130 μm [5].

Most WSL appear on the buccal surface of the tooth, more frequently in male population. Patients who undergo fixed orthodontic treatment show a higher prevalence of WSL, due to the retentive nature of the brackets, wires, and the inherent difficulties in maintaining proper oral hygiene. In orthodontic patients, WSL may appear as soon as 1 month after commencing the treatment, and their incidence is strongly correlated with the duration of the orthodontic therapy. Teeth with lingual brackets are less vulnerable to WLS compared to labial ones, the most important explanation being the much abundant salivary flow [10].

WSL appears as opaque, milky, porous areas, which reflect the light in a different manner when compared to natural translucent enamel. In some cases, WSL may become evident only after drying [7].

Beside visual diagnosis, quantitative light-induced fluorescence (QLF) is an efficient diagnosis method, based on the auto-fluorescence of the tooth when exposed to high-intensity blue light. Being in close relation with the mineral composition of the enamel, low fluorescence is exhibited by demineralized areas. QLF is a much more sensitive method of WSL detection, compared to visual inspection, higher WSL prevalence has been reported by studies using QLF [11].

A proper diagnosis of demineralization-induced WSL has to be carried out by making the differential diagnosis between similar conditions such as developmental enamel defects, and active or inactive carious lesions [10].

## 4. Prevention

Probably the best strategy is to prevent dental biofilm accumulation and improve enamel remineralization. Because of its multifactorial etiology, several approaches have been considered. However, selecting the best prevention method has to be patient-orientated.

### 4.1 Proper oral hygiene

Prevention must commence with educating the patient in maintaining proper oral hygiene, by explaining its importance and complications which, most probably occur in case of poor hygiene. So, detailed instructions are of utmost importance in educating patients on how to maintain adequate oral hygiene. In case of orthodontic patients, instruction should focus on how to clean around brackets. The correct brushing technique, either manual or electric must be explained, and the use of dental floss and mouthwashes must be encouraged. High fluoride concentration toothpastes are being recommended. Electric toothbrushes may represent a particular benefit to patients with higher plaque index. Antiseptic mouthwashes, particularly fluoride and chlorhexidine-based, turned out to be efficient in lowering the *Streptococcus mutans* content. Regular professional cleaning, including scaling, root planning, and topical fluoride application must be more frequent in high-risk patients (every 3 months rather than every 6 months) [12].

### 4.2 Remineralization

Fluoride ions are efficient in preventing demineralization by inhibiting the enzymatic processes involved in bacterial metabolism, and thus inhibiting acid production. A decreased demineralization results in increased remineralization potential, and prevents excessive mineral loss and subsequent caries. Fluoride toothpastes and mouthwashes are meant for daily home use, while periodic topical application of fluoride varnishes, gels, and foams is mainly carried out by the dentist, more frequently in high-risk patients than in low/normal risk cases. Toothpastes with higher fluoride concentrations (1500–5000 ppm) have been shown to have a greater ability to inhibit demineralization and promote remineralization compared to conventional fluoride toothpastes (1000 ppm) [13].

Because the availability of calcium and phosphate ions limits the fluoride accumulation and the remineralization potential of saliva, the preventive efficacy of fluoride alone is questionable. The research toward caries prevention has led to the introduction of CPP-ACP, which is an amorphous form of calcium phosphate (ACP) stabilized by a phosphopeptide from the milk-protein casein (CPP). CPP-ACP has the potential to both prevent demineralization and promote enamel remineralization, by binding to the bacterial wall and, in case of an acid attack, it releases calcium and phosphate ions and maintains a saturation state of the enamel. The presence of CPP at the tooth surface has a certain role in reducing the adhesion of *Streptococcus mutans* and inhibiting bacterial colonization. CPP-ACP containing gels, varnishes, mousses, and chewing gums, with or without fluoride content, are currently available for current use [14].

### 4.3 Diet

A high-carb diet and frequent exposure to fermentable and refined carbohydrates, including sugared beverages, result in a higher risk of developing WSL. This type of beverage not only acts as a nourishing source to acidogenic bacteria but also carries an acid pH of 2–3. As demineralization begins to occur when the pH drops below 5.5, the combination of high sugar content and low pH promotes WSL appearance [15].

Probiotics have shown a great potential to positively impact the oral environment, by reducing the acidogenic microflora and replacing it with non-cariogenic bacterial types [16].

Polyol carbohydrates, such as xylitol, which are non-cariogenic, as they cannot be metabolized by *Streptococcus mutans*, are also involved in reducing the carious risk. By replacing sugar with xylitol in chewing gums, the prevention of bacterial attachment is also carried out by stimulating the salivary flow. Not only physical mechanisms are involved, but stimulated saliva also shows higher phosphate and calcium concentrations [17].

## 5. Treatment

In demineralization-induced WSL, conservative treatment methods such as remineralization, microabrasion, tooth whitening, and resin infiltration are being considered as the first choice. Depending on the case, other therapeutic choices, such as resin restorations and veneers may be necessary, or combined therapy may be attempted.

### 5.1 Remineralization

Remineralization is a non-invasive treatment method, carried out by using fluoride, calcium, and phosphate products. Fluoride, besides caries prevention, and enamel strengthening is also effective in reversing initial, non-cavitated lesions. Applied as varnish or other product forms, fluoride does not show immediate esthetic results, and it needs repeated applications for a certain period of time.

CPP-ACP, combined or not with fluoride, has shown to be effective in preventing and treating WSL. CPP-ACP products also help managing tooth sensitivity [6].

Self-assembling peptides (SAP) are involved in biomimetic enamel remineralization. They are involved in saliva-mediated hydroxyapatite regeneration, by providing additional nucleation sites for the crystallization of salivary calcium and phosphate ions. The most frequently used product is SAP P11-4 (Curodont Repair, Credentis), which has been proven to be effective in treating WSL, alone or associated with fluoride. The SAP P11-4 monomeric solution diffuses into the body of the lesion, and, by promoting new hydroxyapatite formation below the porous mineralized surface, it results in reducing the size of the WSL [18–20].

### 5.2 Microabrasion

Microabrasion is usually carried out by combining chemical erosion, using acid solutions such as HCl, and mechanical abrasion using pumice stones or brushes. HCl action consists of the decontamination and removal of the affected enamel areas and enhances the subsequent mechanical treatment. This method is considered to be safe and effective, especially in small WSL (< 0.2 mm diameter), and in combination with tooth whitening [21].

### 5.3 Tooth whitening

Tooth whitening is a minimally invasive technique, widely used in treating tooth discolorations. In case of WSL, after whitening, their milky appearance blends with the enhanced luminosity of the bleached unaffected tooth substance. The shade difference between the WSL and the sound enamel usually decreases, however, sometimes, the result may not be the expected one, and the WSL may look even worse after whitening. Whitening is especially indicated in old, inactive WSL [19, 22].

### 5.4 Resin infiltration

Resin infiltration is a microinvasive treatment option, an alternative to microabrasion, and it involves pretreating the WSL by using HCl, followed by subsequent infiltration with a low-viscosity light-cured resin, without mechanical removal of the surface layer. The acid leaves the tubules open, prepared for resin infiltration [23].

The white, chalky appearance of WSL is due to an optical phenomenon, caused by the difference between the refraction indexes of sound enamel and the porous, demineralized lesion. Because of hydroxyapatite dissolution, microspaces full of liquid and air were left behind. The idea was of filling these voids with a low-viscosity resin, capable of penetrating the microporosities of the etched enamel. As the infiltrating resin has a similar refraction index to hydroxyapatite, the human eye will perceive the tooth as being sound. Resin infiltration results in immediate improved esthetics and does not limit other dental treatments [22].

Resin microinfiltration results in increased microhardness, when compared to untreated or remineralized WSL, which leads to better fracture and abrasion resistance, comprehensive strength, and elasticity. This feature is due to the fact that the low-viscosity resin fills the pores and creates a diffusion barrier at the surface and within the inner part of the lesion. Thus, a re-hardening of the demineralized tooth structure takes place [24].

Regarding penetration efficiency, opposite opinions may be found in the literature. Some studies claim that the depth penetration is good, while other studies argue that the hypermineralized surface layer of early carious lesions may prevent the proper penetration of the infiltrating resin, despite the initial surface treatment using 15% HCl, questioning its efficacy and restricting it to the enamel surface [25–28].

## 6. WSL treatment using resin infiltration: some case reports

The most frequently used and efficient resin infiltration product, widely studied since its release on the market, is the ICON kit (DMG, Hamburg, Germany) [29].

Resin infiltration treatment of WSL by using the ICON kit (Infiltration CONcept) is a microinvasive, well-tolerated method, with immediate results. ICON is recognized as effective in enhancing esthetics and reducing the risk of caries progression, thus avoiding or postponing the necessity for more extensive restorative approaches, thus having a protective-preventive role [30, 31].

The enamel structure is characterized by the presence of microporosities, which allows the low-viscosity resin to penetrate the depth of the affected enamel, filling all the voids, and resulting in the modification of its refraction index, as the resin has the same optic properties as sound enamel [30].

The system is based on three components (**Figure 1**): ICON-Etch (HCl 15%), ICON-Dry (ethanol), and ICON-Infiltrant (TEGDMA-based, low-viscosity light-cured resin). Its indication extends to treating incipient caries in both adults and children, being patient-friendly, as it does not involve rotary instrumentation or anesthesia [31, 32]. As it works on the infiltration principle, a dry field is necessary, and using rubber dam is required. The rubber dam also protects the soft tissues from the action of HCl, which may cause chemical burns. In order to gain a dry environment, ICON-dry (ethanol) is used to enable water evaporation from the porosities [31].

The technique involves etching with HCl 15%, 2 minutes, washing, drying with an air syringe, 30 seconds, ethanol application, injecting the resin, followed by light-curing. The process should be closely monitorized, as the ICON-dry application outlines if the enamel area to be infiltrated has been properly demineralized. If the enamel discoloration does not show significant improvement after one application of ICON-etch and ICON-dry, the manufacturer advises repetition, up to a maximum of three applications [32].

This is the case of hypermineralized enamel, where more than one ICON-Etch and ICON-Dry application is frequently necessary, in the attempt to penetrate the superficial

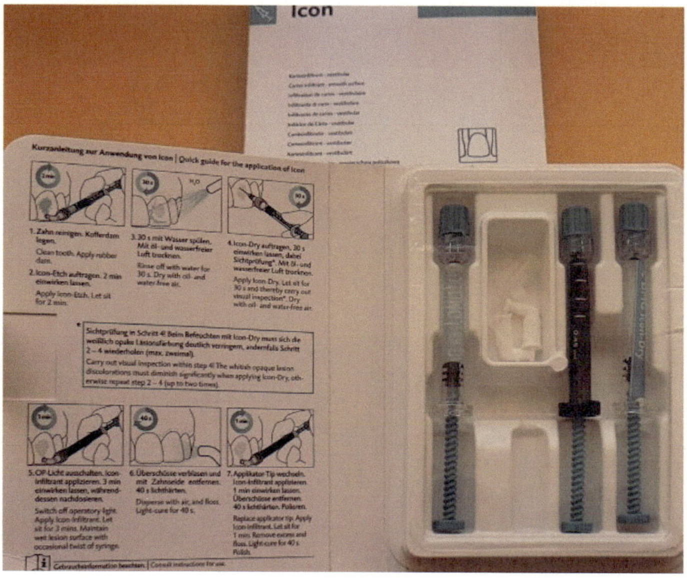


**Figure 1.**
*The ICON kit (DMG (Hamburg, Germany)).*

layer and reach the underlying area, which still displays microporosities, and thus being characterized by a different refraction index compared with sound surrounding areas [31].

In order to illustrate the immediate esthetic outcome of ICON in treating WSL, three cases of different etiology and age were selected.

### 6.1 Case 1

Case 1: WSL due to fixed orthodontic treatment, which appeared 1.5 years prior to ICON treatment. WSL were localized on 1.1, 1.2, 1.3, 2.1, 2.2, and 2.3 labial side (**Figure 2**). In this case, three applications (which is the maximum prescribed by the manufacturer) of ICON-Etch and ICON-Dry were carried out.

The treatment results are visible and may be described as follows: 1.1-complete blur of 80% of the area (**Figures 3** and **4**); 1.2-complete blur of 95% of the area (**Figure 4**);

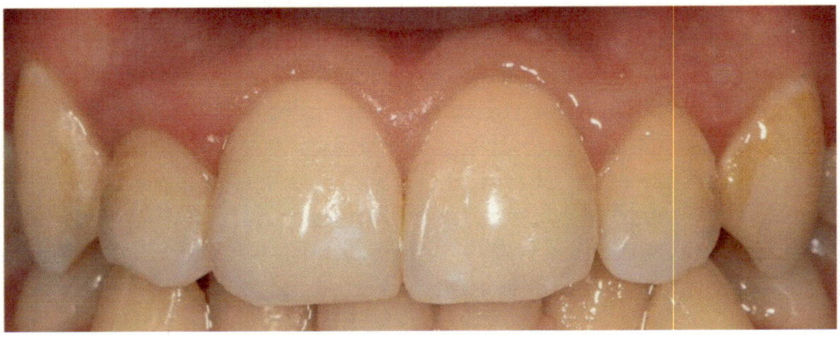

**Figure 2.**
*Case 1, WSL localized at 1.1, 1.2, 1.3, 2.1, 2.2, 2.3.*

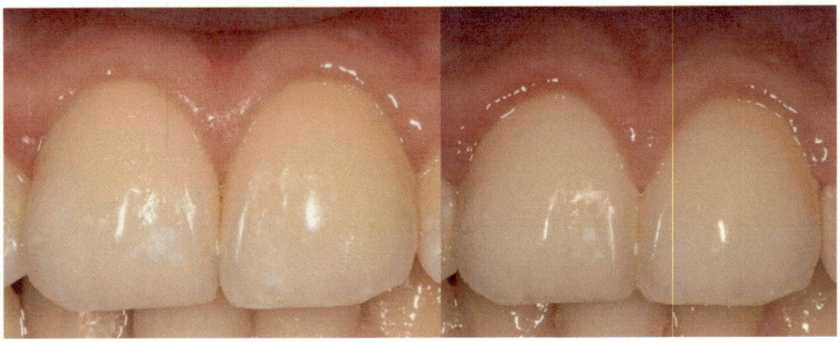

**Figure 3.**
*Case 1, 1.1 and 2.1 before and after treatment.*

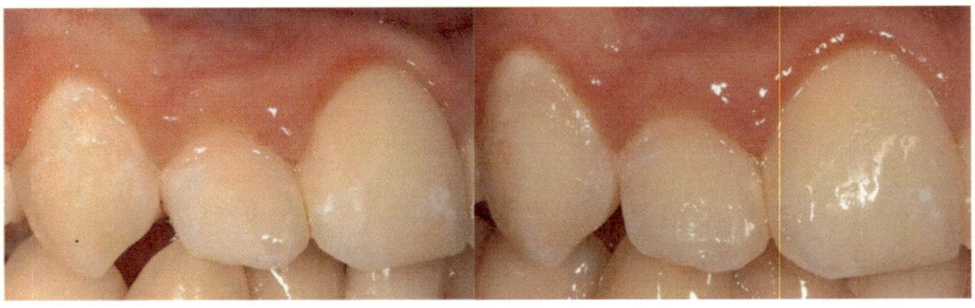

**Figure 4.**
*Case 1, 1.1, 1.2, and 1.3 before and after treatment.*

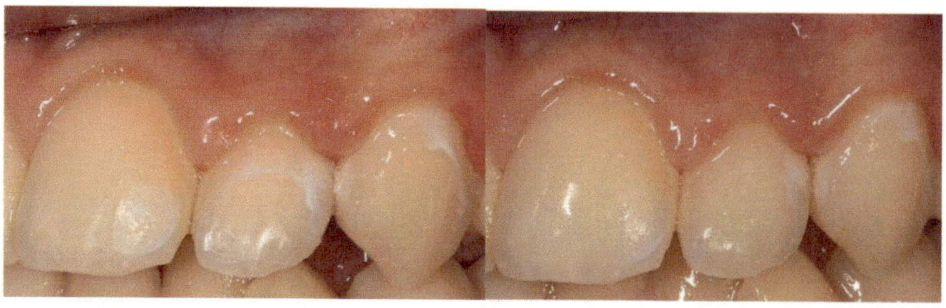

**Figure 5.**
*Case 1, 2.1, 2.2, and 2.3 before and after treatment.*

1.3-complete blur of 50% of the area, the rest being partially blurred (**Figure 4**); 2.1-mesial WSL-partial blur of the entire area; distal WSL-almost complete blur of 90% of the area (**Figures 3** and **5**); 2.2-complete blur of 70% of the area (**Figure 5**); 2.3-no improvement (**Figure 5**).

### 6.2 Case 2

Case 2: WSL due to fixed orthodontic treatment, relatively new (appeared several months prior to ICON treatment). The orthodontic device was removed 1 week prior to ICON treatment. WSL were localized in the upper part of the labial surface of 1.1, 1.2, 2.1, 2.2, 2.3 (**Figure 6**). Only one application of ICON-Etch and ICON-Dry was carried out. In case of 1.1, 2.1 there's complete resolution, 1.2 shows 80% complete blur, and 2.2, 2.3 show 90% complete blur (**Figure 7**).

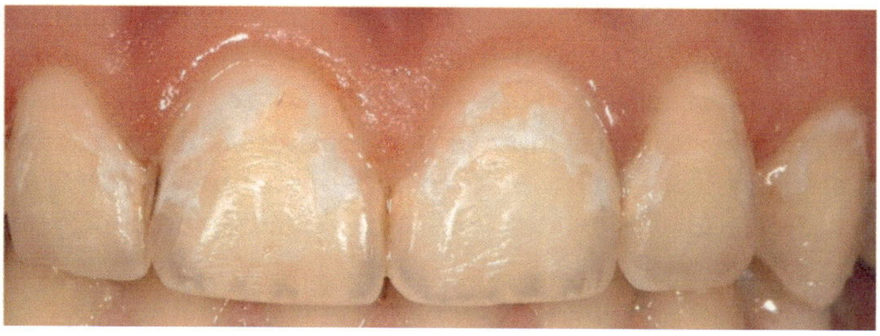

**Figure 6.**
*Case 2, WSL localized at 1.1, 1.2, 2.1, 2.2, 2.3.*

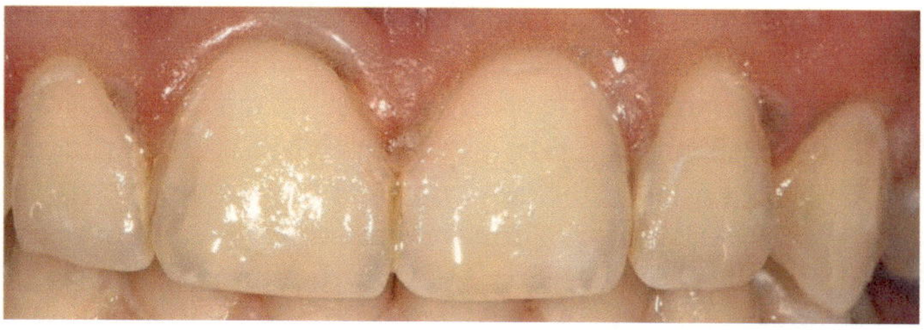

**Figure 7.**
*Case 2, Posttreatment image.*

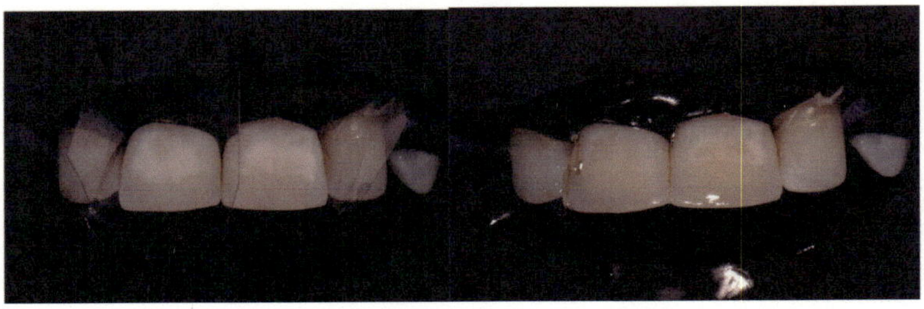

**Figure 8.**
*Case 3, before and after treatment.*

## 6.3 Case 3

Case 3: non-orthodontic patient, with past neglected oral hygiene. After the occurrence of WSL, 2 years prior ICON treatment, the patient had improved oral hygiene, but there was no change. WSL were localized in the central part of the labial side of 1.1, 1.2 (**Figure 8**), and three applications of ICON-Etch and ICON-Dry were carried out. After treatment a complete blur of 75% of the area was seen in 1.1, and 50% in 2.1 (**Figure 8**).

Despite the fact that the post-treatment images of the three cases illustrated still show signs of milky areas, the patients were completely satisfied with the outcome, as their entourage no longer observes the issue.

## 7. Discussion

When referring to which is the most effective or the most frequently used treatment for WSL, the data found in the literature are quite controversial.

According to Saito, the most frequent treatment for WSL is fluoride, namely prescription of 5000 ppm toothpaste, followed by fluoride varnish and mouthwash [33]. Weiland also states that fluoride is the first choice of therapy in orthodontic patients, after bracket removal, followed by resin infiltration, microabrasion, resin fillings, veneers, no therapy, and tooth whitening [7]. According to Guzman, no treatment in the first 6 months after debonding may allow natural remineralization to take place, without any intervention. If this is not the case, the extent of the lesion and the urge for esthetic rehabilitation should be considered when deciding the treatment [34]. Sonnenson states that natural remineralization and tooth brushing twice a day with fluoride toothpaste may be the first option after debonding, followed by close monitoring for 3–6 months [35].

Despite the fact that fluoride is the most frequently prescribed for WSL treatment, systematic reviews by Sardana [36], Hu [37], and Sonesson [35] concluded that there's no reliable information to support the effectiveness of topical remineralizing agents (fluoride and CPP-ACP) in treating post-orthodontic WSL. According to Sonnenson, fluoride in high concentrations (fluoride varnishes) may interfere with natural remineralization, due to surface hypermineralization, and result in permanent brown staining, with esthetic consequences [35]. On the other hand, SAPs are being mentioned as having promising results in both demineralization prevention and enamel remineralization. Using SAP P11-4 in combination with fluoride was shown to be more effective than fluoride alone [18, 38–40].

Akin compared the outcome of microabrasion with HCl and pumice to tooth brushing and concluded that microabrasion had a better outcome over a 6-month period [41]. Gu compared the esthetic effect of microabrasion and resin infiltration, over a 12-months period, and concluded that both showed sufficient durability, with a better outcome in case of resin infiltration [42]. According to Sonnensen, microabrasion and resin infiltration are efficient in more severe cases of post-orthodontic WSLs, but their disadvantage is being technique-sensitive. Microabrasion has to be repeated several times, while resin infiltration is a single-appointment treatment, but up to three rounds of etching may be needed [35].

Resin infiltration is an alternative to both prevent the WSL progression, with subsequent cavity formation and improvement of the esthetic appearance. The esthetic results in the case of anterior WSL may not be perfect, but resin infiltration has shown immediately improved esthetical appearance, when compared to untreated lesions, as well as good durability in short or long-term follow-ups. A study by Knosel considers that, after a 20-month follow-up, the assimilation of resin-infiltrated WSL to the color of adjacent teeth is suitable for a long-term esthetic improvement [43]. A meta-analysis conducted by Bouroni states that resin infiltration shows better esthetic results compared to fluoride varnish, much more, the effect of fluoride shows after several regular applications, which may take up to 6 months [26]. A recent study by Ibrahim concluded that both fluoride and resin infiltration improve the esthetic appearance of WSL, but resin infiltration lasts longer [27]. According to several systematic reviews, resin infiltration of WSL is effective in inhibiting further caries progression, in both primary and permanent teeth. Resin infiltration has proven to be more effective than the no-treatment approach and non-invasive methods such as fluoride varnish application, or hygiene instruction [25, 44]. A study by Urquhart states that the combination of resin infiltration and 5% sodium fluoride varnish is 5 times more efficient in WSL treatment, compared to no treatment [45]. Several systematic and umbrella reviews confirm the ability of resin infiltration to inhibit WSL and non-cavitated proximal enamel lesions progression, the relative risk of subsequent caries development being substantially diminished [25, 29, 44–46]. According to Cebula [29], long-term monitoring of lesion progression was confirmed by recent studies, follow-ups being usually carried out at 12–48 months, depending on the study [47–50], or even at 7 years in a study conducted by Paris [30].

The 3 cases described in Section 6 are of different etiology and age. Two cases (Case 1 and 2) were of post-orthodontic treatment WSL and one of a non-orthodontic patient (case 3), with past neglected oral hygiene. The WSL of case 2 were quite new (several months prior ICON treatment), while the WSL of case 1 and 3 were older (more than 1 year prior treatment). In Case 2, only one application of ICON-Etch and ICON-Dry was necessary, while in Cases 1 and 3, the maximum of three applications of ICON-Etch and ICON-Dry were needed. In Case 2, out of the five WSL, two showed complete resolution, one showed 80% complete blur, and two showed 90% complete blur. In Cases 1 and 3, which exhibited older WSL, out of a total of eight lesions, one showed no improvement, six showed complete blur of 50–95% of the area, one was only partially blurred, and one showed complete blur of 50% of the area, the rest is partially blurred.

The better immediate esthetic outcome, with almost complete resolution of the WSL after only one application, has been observed in case of more recent lesions (Case 2). This may be explained by the still present large structural porosities, which allow the resin to penetrate the depth of the affected enamel, thus filling all the voids, and resulting in the modification of the refraction index. In case of older and deeper WSL, three ICON-Etch and ICON-Dry applications were necessary, in the attempt to penetrate the superficial remineralized enamel layer, and to reach the underlying area, which still displays voids, and thus being characterized by a different refraction index compared with sound surrounding areas. In cases of older lesions, no complete resolution was obtained, but the esthetic results were still encouraging and the patients were completely satisfied with the treatment outcome. This result is in line with previously published articles, which state that new, shallow lesions needed only one infiltration step, with good esthetic outcome, while older and deeper lesions were only partially masked after several applications [31, 51].

## 8. Conclusion

The treatment method in case of demineralization-induced WSL depends on the extent and esthetic gravity of the lesion and should be selected only after attempting the no treatment and at-home care options, in cases where these show to be inefficient. The resin infiltration method has good immediate results, and according to recent studies, has been proven to be not only esthetically suitable but also efficient in preventing the lesion progression, with long-term promising results.

## Acknowledgements

The authors wish to express their thanks to Dr. Gloria Golban for her valuable contribution.

## Conflict of interest

The authors declare no conflict of interest.

## Author details

Lavinia Cosmina Ardelean[1]*, Codruta Victoria Tigmeanu[1], Alexandra Roi[2] and Laura-Cristina Rusu[2]

1 Department of Technology of Materials and Devices in Dental Medicine, Multidisciplinary Center for Research, Evaluation, Diagnosis and Therapies in Oral Medicine, "Victor Babeş" University of Medicine and Pharmacy Timisoara, Timisoara, Romania

2 Department of Oral Pathology, Multidisciplinary Center for Research, Evaluation, Diagnosis and Therapies in Oral Medicine, "Victor Babeş" University of Medicine and Pharmacy Timisoara, Timisoara, Romania

*Address all correspondence to: lavinia_ardelean@umft.ro

## References

[1] Etiology and Management of White Spot Lesions. 2016. Available from: https://decisionsindentistry.com/article/lesions-0116/ [Accessed: April 26, 2024]

[2] Nota A, Palumbo L, Pantaleo G, Gherlone EF, Tecco S. Developmental enamel defects (DDE) and their association with oral health, preventive procedures, and children's psychosocial attitudes towards home oral hygiene: A cross-sectional study. International Journal of Environmental Research and Public Health. 2020;**17**:4025. DOI: 10.3390/ijerph17114025

[3] de Farias AL, Rojas-Gualdrón DF, Girotto Bussaneli D, Santos-Pinto L, Mejía JD, Restrepo M. Does molar-incisor hypomineralization (MIH) affect only permanent first molars and incisors? New observations on permanent second molars. International Journal of Paediatric Dentistry. 2022;**32**:1-10. DOI: 10.1111/ipd.12780

[4] Vélez-León E, Albaladejo-Martínez A, Pacheco-Quito EM, Armas-Vega A, Delgado-Gaete A, Pesántez-Ochoa D, et al. Developmental enamel defects in children from the southern region of Ecuador. Children (Basel). 2022;**9**:1755. DOI: 10.3390/children9111755

[5] Fejerskov O, Nyvad B, editors. Dental Caries: The Disease and its Clinical Management. 4th ed. Chichester, UK: Wiley; 2024. 9 p

[6] Lopes PC, Carvalho T, Gomes ATPC, Veiga N, Blanco L, Correia MJ, et al. White spot lesions: Diagnosis and treatment—A systematic review. BMC Oral Health. 2024;**24**:58. DOI: 10.1186/s12903-023-03720-6

[7] Weyland MI, Jost-Brinkmann PG, Bartzela T. Management of white spot lesions induced during orthodontic treatment with multibracket appliance: A national-based survey. Clinical Oral Investigations. 2022;**26**:4871-4883. DOI: 10.1007/s00784-022-04454-5

[8] Chen X, Daliri EB, Kim N, Kim JR, Yoo D, Oh DH. Microbial etiology and prevention of dental caries: Exploiting natural products to inhibit cariogenic biofilms. Pathogens. 2020;**9**:569. DOI: 10.3390/pathogens9070569

[9] Lemos JA, Palmer SR, Zeng L, Wen ZT, Kajfasz JK, Freires IA, et al. The biology of *Streptococcus mutans*. Microbiology Spectrum. 2019;**7**:1128. DOI: 10.1128/microbiolspec.GPP3-0051-2018

[10] Marinelli G, Inchingolo AD, Inchingolo AM, Malcangi G, Limongelli L, Montenegro V, et al. White spot lesions in orthodontics: Prevention and treatment. A descriptive review. Journal of Biological Regulators and Homeostatic Agents. 2021;**35**:227-240. DOI: 10.23812/21-2supp1-24

[11] Oh SH, Choi JY, Kim SH. Evaluation of dental caries detection with quantitative light-induced fluorescence in comparison to different field of view devices. Scientific Reports. 2022;**12**:6139. DOI: 10.1038/s41598-022-10126-x

[12] Guo J, Li L, Guan G, Bennani F, Mei L. Oral health knowledge and practice among orthodontic clients in China and New Zealand. Canadian Journal Of Dental Hygiene. 2020;**1**:124-132

[13] Simmer JP, Hardy NC, Chinoy AF, Bartlett JD, Hu JC. How fluoride protects dental enamel from demineralization. Journal of International Society of

Preventive and Community Dentistry. 2020;**10**:134-141. DOI: 10.4103/jispcd.JISPCD_406_19

[14] Sionov RV, Tsavdaridou D, Aqawi M, Zaks B, Steinberg D, Shalish M. Tooth mousse containing casein phosphopeptide-amorphous calcium phosphate prevents biofilm formation of *Streptococcus mutans*. BMC Oral Health. 2021;**21**:136. DOI: 10.1186/s12903-021-01502-6

[15] Mahboobi Z, Pakdaman A, Yazdani R, Azadbakht L, Montazeri A. Dietary free sugar and dental caries in children: A systematic review on longitudinal studies. Health Promotion Perspective. 2021;**11**:271-280. DOI: 10.34172/hpp.2021.35

[16] Butt S, Sin M. Can probiotics prevent dental caries? Evidence-Based Dentistry. 2023;**24**:130-131. DOI: 10.1038/s41432-023-00918-z

[17] ALHumaid J, Bamashmous M. Meta-analysis on the effectiveness of xylitol in caries prevention. Journal of International Society of Preventive and Community Dentistry 2022;12:133-138DOI: 10.4103/jispcd.JISPCD_164_21

[18] Sedlakova Kondelova P, Mannaa A, Bommer C, Abdelaziz M, Daeniker L, di Bella E, et al. Efficacy of $P_{11}$-4 for the treatment of initial buccal caries: A randomized clinical trial. Scientific Reports. 2020;**10**:20211. DOI: 10.1038/s41598-020-77057-3

[19] Roig-Vanaclocha A, Solá-Ruiz MF, Román-Rodríguez JL, Amengual-Lorenzo J, Alonso Pérez-Barquero J, Agustín-Panadero R. Dental treatment of white spots and a description of the technique and digital quantification of the loss of enamel volume. Applied Sciences. 2020;**10**:4369. DOI: 10.3390/app10124369

[20] Nath SJC, Fu Y, Li KC, Loho T, Loch C, Ekambaram M. A comparison of the enamel remineralisation potential of self-assembling peptides. International Dental Journal. 2023;**S0020-6539**(23):00123-00125. DOI: 10.1016/j.identj.2023.07.003

[21] Román-Rodríguez JL, Agustín-Panadero R, Roig-Vanaclocha A, Amengual-Lorenzo J. A tooth whitening and chemical abrasive protocol for the treatment of developmental enamel defects. The Journal of Prosthetic Dentistry. 2020;**123**:379-383. DOI: 10.1016/j.prosdent.2019.02.015

[22] Tajmehr N. A minimally invasive treatment for white spots on teeth. BDJ Team. 2020;7:20-23. DOI: 10.1038/s41407-019-0212-5

[23] Allen DN, Fine CM, Newton MN, Kabani F, Muzzin KB, Reed KM. Resin infiltration therapy: A micro-invasive treatment approach for white spot lesions. Journal of Dental Hygiene. 2021;**95**:31-35

[24] Zakizade M, Davoudi A, Akhavan A, Shirban F. Effect of resin infiltration technique on improving surface hardness of enamel lesions: A systematic review and meta-analysis. The Journal of Evidence-Based Dental Practice. 2020;**20**:101405. DOI: 10.1016/j.jebdp.2020.101405

[25] Lin GSS, Chan DZK, Lee HY, Low TT, Laer TS, Pillai MPM, et al. Effectiveness of resin infiltration in caries inhibition and aesthetic appearance improvement of white-spot lesions: An umbrella review. The Journal of Evidence-Based Dental Practice. 2022;**22**:101723. DOI: 10.1016/j.jebdp.2022.101723

[26] Bourouni S, Dritsas K, Kloukos D, Wierichs RJ. Efficacy of resin infiltration

to mask post-orthodontic or non-post-orthodontic white spot lesions or fluorosis—A systematic review and meta-analysis. Clinical Oral Investigations. 2021;**25**:4711-4719. DOI: 10.1007/s00784-021-03931-7

[27] Ibrahim DFA, Venkiteswaran A, Hasmun NN. Esthetic effects and color stability of resin infiltration on demineralized enamel lesions: A systematic review. Journal of International Society of Preventive and Community Dentistry. 2023;**13**:273-286. DOI: 10.4103/jispcd.JISPCD_29_23

[28] Dziaruddin N, Zakaria ASI. Resin infiltration of non-cavitated enamel lesions in paediatric dentistry: A narrative review. Children (Basel). 2022;**9**:1893. DOI: 10.3390/children9121893

[29] Cebula M, Göstemeyer G, Krois J, Pitchika V, Paris S, Schwendicke F, et al. Resin infiltration of non-cavitated proximal caries lesions in primary and permanent teeth: A systematic review and scenario analysis of randomized controlled trials. Journal of Clinical Medicine. 2023;**12**:727. DOI: 10.3390/jcm12020727

[30] Paris S, Bitter K, Krois J, Meyer-Lueckel H. Seven-year-efficacy of proximal caries infiltration—Randomized clinical trial. Journal of Dentistry. 2020;**93**:103277. DOI: 10.1016/j.jdent.2020.103277

[31] Ibrahim DFA, Liew YM, Hasmun NN, Venkiteswaran A. Resin infiltration ICON: A guide for clinical use. Malaysian Journal of Pediatric Dentistry. 2023;**2**:27-35

[32] Tavares MI, Saraiva J, do Vale F, Coelho AS, Amaro IF, Marto CM, et al. Resin infiltration in white spot lesions caused by orthodontic hypomineralisation: A minimally invasive therapy. British Dental Journal. 2021;**231**:387-392. DOI: 10.1038/s41415-021-3476-z

[33] Saito T, Park JH, Bay C. A survey of pediatric dentists on the treatment timing and modalities for white spot lesions in the United States. The Journal of Clinical Pediatric Dentistry. 2019;**43**:27-33. DOI: 10.17796/1053-4625-43.1.6

[34] Guzman-Armstrong S, Chalmers J, Warren JJ, Ask us. White spot lesions: Prevention and treatment. American Journal of Orthodontics and Dentofacial Orthopedics. 2010;**138**:690-696. DOI: 10.1016/j.ajodo.2010.07.007

[35] Sonesson M, Bergstrand F, Gizani S, Twetman S. Management of post-orthodontic white spot lesions: An updated systematic review. European Journal of Orthodontics. 2017;**39**:116-121. DOI: 10.1093/ejo/cjw023

[36] Sardana D, Zhang J, Ekambaram M, Yang Y, McGrath CP, Yiu CKY. Effectiveness of professional fluorides against enamel white spot lesions during fixed orthodontic treatment: A systematic review and meta-analysis. Journal of Dentistry. 2019;**82**:1-10. DOI: 10.1016/j.jdent.2018.12.006

[37] Hu H, Feng C, Jiang Z, Wang L, Shrestha S, Yan J, et al. Effectiveness of remineralizing agents in the prevention and reversal of orthodontically induced white spot lesions: A systematic review and network meta-analysis. Clinical Oral Investigations. 2020;**24**:4153-4167. DOI: 10.1007/s00784-020-03610-z

[38] Jablonski-Momeni A, Nothelfer R, Morawietz M, Kiesow A, Korbmacher-Steiner H. Impact of self-assembling peptides in remineralisation of artificial early enamel lesions adjacent

to orthodontic brackets. Scientific Reports. 2020;**10**:15132. DOI: 10.1038/s41598-020-72185-2

[39] Doberdoli D, Bommer C, Begzati A, et al. Randomized clinical trial investigating self-assembling peptide $P_{11}$-4 for treatment of early occlusal caries. Scientific Reports. 2020;**10**:4195. DOI: 10.1038/s41598-020-60815-8

[40] Welk A, Ratzmann A, Reich M, Krey KF, Schwahn C. Effect of self-assembling peptide $P_{11}$-4 on orthodontic treatment-induced carious lesions. Scientific Reports. 2020;**10**:6819. DOI: 10.1038/s41598-020-63633-0

[41] Akin M, Basciftci FA. Can white spot lesions be treated effectively? The Angle Orthodontist. 2012;**82**:770-775. DOI: 10.2319/090711.578.1

[42] Gu X, Yang L, Yang D, Gao Y, Duan X, Zhu X, et al. Esthetic improvements of postorthodontic white-spot lesions treated with resin infiltration and microabrasion: A split-mouth, randomized clinical trial. The Angle Orthodontist. 2019;**89**:372-377. DOI: 10.2319/041218-274.1

[43] Knösel M, Eckstein A, Helms HJ. Long-term follow-up of camouflage effects following resin infiltration of post orthodontic white-spot lesions in vivo. The Angle Orthodontist. 2019;**89**:33-39. DOI: 10.2319/052118-383.1

[44] Tedesco TK, Calvo AFB, Pássaro AL, Araujo MP, Ladewig NM, Scarpini S, et al. Non restorative treatment of initial caries lesion in primary teeth: A systematic review and network meta-analysis. Acta Odontologica Scandinavica. 2022;**80**:1-8. DOI: 10.1080/00016357.2021.1928748

[45] Urquhart O, Tampi MP, Pilcher L, Slayton RL, Araujo MWB, Fontana M, et al. Nonrestorative treatments for caries: Systematic review and network meta-analysis. Journal of Dental Research. 2019;**98**:14-26. DOI: 10.1177/0022034518800014

[46] Chen Y, Chen D, Lin H. Infiltration and sealing for managing non-cavitated proximal lesions: A systematic review and meta-analysis. BMC Oral Health. 2021;**21**:13. DOI: 10.1186/s12903-020-01364-4

[47] Meyer-Lueckel H, Wardius A, Krois J, Bitter K, Moser C, Paris S, et al. Proximal caries infiltration—Pragmatic RCT with 4 years of follow-up. Journal of Dentistry. 2021;**111**:103733. DOI: 10.1016/j.jdent.2021.103733

[48] Arslan S, Kaplan MH. The effect of resin infiltration on the progression of proximal caries lesions: A randomized clinical trial. Medical Principles and Practice. 2020;**29**:238-243. DOI: 10.1159/000503053

[49] Peters MC, Hopkins AR Jr, Zhu L, Yu Q. Efficacy of proximal resin infiltration on caries inhibition: Results from a 3-year randomized controlled clinical trial. Journal of Dental Research. 2019;**98**:1497-1502. DOI: 10.1177/0022034519876853

[50] Sarti CS, Vizzotto MB, Filgueiras LV, Bonifácio CC, Rodrigues JA. Two-year split-mouth randomized controlled clinical trial on the progression of proximal carious lesions on primary molars after resin infiltration. Pediatric Dentistry. 2020;**42**:110-115

[51] Abbas BA, Marzouk ES, Zaher AR. Treatment of various degrees of white spot lesions using resin infiltration-in vitro study. Progress in Orthodontics. 2018;**19**:27. DOI: 10.1186/s40510-018-0223-3

Chapter 6

# Dentin-Pulp Interaction with Silver Diamine Fluoride

*Divya Mudumba*

## Abstract

Silver diamine fluoride (SDF) is increasingly used as a non-invasive treatment modality for caries management, particularly in pediatric and geriatric populations. Understanding its impact on the dentin-pulp complex is crucial for assessing its efficacy and safety in preserving pulp health while arresting carious lesions. SDF application directly affects the dentin-pulp complex by interacting with dentin, potentially influencing pulp health and function. Exploring how SDF interacts with dentin and its effects on pulp tissue would provide valuable insights into the dentin-pulp complex. Also, dentists and clinicians need to be aware of the potential effects of SDF on the dentin-pulp complex when considering its use in caries management protocols. Discussing clinical considerations, such as indications, contraindications, application techniques, and patient selection criteria, would be valuable for dental practitioners.

**Keywords:** silver diamine fluoride, preventive dentistry, caries management, cariology, minimal intervention dentistry

## 1. Introduction

Silver diamine fluoride (SDF) has emerged as a valuable tool in contemporary dentistry, particularly for its unique properties in arresting dental caries and managing hypersensitivity. This innovative solution, composed of silver, fluoride, and ammonia, presents a non-invasive approach to caries management, especially in populations where traditional restorative interventions may be challenging or impractical.

Beyond its antimicrobial and remineralizing properties, SDF has gained attention for its efficacy in managing dentin hypersensitivity, a common complaint among patients. The application of SDF results in the formation of a silver protein layer over exposed dentin tubules, effectively blocking the transmission of stimuli that cause sensitivity, thereby providing relief to patients.

In recent years, SDF has garnered significant interest due to its simplicity of application, cost-effectiveness, and potential to improve oral health outcomes, particularly in underserved communities and pediatric populations. However, despite its promise, concerns persist regarding its esthetic impact, potential discoloration, and long-term effects on dental tissues, especially the dental pulp.

Understanding the interaction between SDF and the dental pulp is crucial for optimizing its clinical application and ensuring patient safety. This chapter aims to explore the chemistry, mechanisms of action, clinical applications, and potential impacts of SDF on dental pulp tissues, shedding light on its role in modern dental practice and guiding evidence-based decision-making.

## 2. Chemistry and mechanism of action of SDF

SDF's mechanism of action is multifaceted. It leverages silver ions to inhibit the growth and metabolism of cariogenic bacteria, thereby halting the progression of dental caries. Fluoride ions contribute to the remineralization of enamel and dentin, promoting the formation of fluorapatite crystals, which enhance the structural integrity of the tooth. This dual action not only arrests decay but also fortifies tooth structure, offering a conservative alternative to conventional restorative treatments.

SDF is a transparent aqueous solution of silver ions and fluoride ions. Unlike silver fluoride (AgF), SDF exhibits a lower alkalinity with a pH ranging between 8 and 9. This characteristic eliminates the need for a reducing agent, simplifying its application process. SDF is recognized for its stability and ability to maintain a consistent concentration over time, making it a preferred choice for caries arrest in various countries, including China and Japan [1]. The longevity of SDF's effectiveness in halting dental caries has been established through years of practical application and research.

Fung et al. [2] proposed that SDF exerts its effects through two primary mechanisms: fluoride ions primarily act on the tooth structure, while the silver phosphate component combats cariogenic bacteria. When applied, SDF interacts with the hydroxyapatite in enamel, resulting in the formation of fluorapatite [Ca10(PO4)6F2], which has demonstrated greater resistance to acidic environments compared to hydroxyapatite. Furthermore, SDF exhibits antimicrobial properties against *Streptococcus mutans* and *Actinomyces naeslundii* on dentin surfaces. Studies have also indicated that SDF inhibits the adherence of biofilms, consequently reducing bacterial colonization on enamel surfaces. The characteristic black-stained layer associated with arrested dentin caries manifests as a durable and impermeable layer of silver phosphate, effectively shielding collagen exposure [3]. These findings underscore the multifaceted nature of SDF's action, highlighting its potential in caries management and microbial control.

Research findings indicate that SDF does not provoke inflammation or necrosis of the dental pulp. Furthermore, studies have demonstrated the potential for SDF to stimulate the formation of tertiary dentin. These observations suggest that SDF holds promise as a viable option for indirect pulp therapy in cases involving deep cavities. This characteristic underscores its potential as a conservative approach to managing deep carious lesions while preserving pulp vitality and promoting dentin repair. However, further research and clinical studies are necessary to validate its efficacy and safety for such applications [4].

## 3. Clinical applications of SDF

SDF serves as a non-invasive treatment option for managing dental caries, alleviating dentin hypersensitivity, and promoting preventive dental care. Its effectiveness, ease of application, and cost-efficiency make it a valuable tool in various clinical scenarios, ranging from pediatric dentistry to geriatric care. The scope of clinical applications of SDF can be divided into the following categories:

### 3.1 Pediatric dentistry

SDF proves to be an effective solution for managing early childhood caries, particularly in cases where children may exhibit challenges in cooperation or understanding, rendering them unsuitable candidates for conventional restorative treatments. Additionally, it offers a practical approach when children present with multiple cavitated lesions, potentially reducing the need for multiple visits to address each lesion individually.

### 3.2 Geriatric dentistry

Older adults often face unique oral health challenges that increase their susceptibility to dental caries. Factors such as exposed root surfaces, periodontal disease, and systemic conditions or medications altering oral flora contribute to their heightened risk. These conditions necessitate tailored dental care approaches to address their specific needs and ensure optimal oral health outcomes. Exposed root dentin resulting from gum recession is susceptible to demineralization at a pH level less acidic than that required for enamel demineralization, exacerbating the risk of dental caries. A substantial portion of tooth decay is attributed to recurrent disease linked with deteriorating restorations. Notably, the majority of dental caries observed in older adults stems from restoration failure specifically at the gingival margin [5]. These lesions can be specifically challenging to restore efficiently.

### 3.3 Special needs

SDF can be used to manage dental caries in patients with special needs who may have difficulty complying with traditional restorative treatments or who require a less invasive approach to dental care. Many special needs patients experience sensory sensitivities or sensory processing disorders. SDF application is quick and minimally invasive, reducing the potential for sensory overload or discomfort during dental visits. Special needs patients often face challenges with oral hygiene maintenance, putting them at a higher risk for dental caries. SDF can be applied preventively to halt the progression of early carious lesions and prevent the need for more extensive dental treatments in the future. In a recommendation by Crystal et al. in 2017, [6] 38% SDF was advocated to be effective in arresting cavitated caries lesions in children and adolescents, including those with special health care needs.

### 3.4 Community health care setting

Dental public health initiatives and programs aim to optimize caries prevention and management strategies that are minimally invasive, safe and simple to administer, affordable, and can be carried out by various members of dental treatment teams [7]. Furthermore, in the context of the widespread transmission of the SARS-CoV-2 virus (COVID-19), SDF has emerged as a recommended caries management procedure that is non-surgical, non-aerosolizing, and aligns with directives from public health authorities, regulatory agencies, and professional organizations aimed at minimizing the risk of airborne pathogen transmission [8]. SDF fulfills all these criteria and recent evidence also indicates the acceptance of SDF among dentally underserved patient groups for its application in posterior dentition. When presented to parents as a safe, minimally invasive, and effective alternative to potentially painful procedures or those requiring sedation for their children, SDF has been favored, especially for children with behavioral challenges [9].

## 4. Interactions of silver diamine fluoride with dentin and dental pulp

### 4.1 Direct effects

#### *4.1.1 Pulpal irritation and cytotoxicity*

In a study by Hosoya et al. direct application of SDF on dental pulp caused severe inflammation and necrosis of dental pulp [10] in most of the teeth in the experimental group. This result was attributed to the high toxicity of silver ions and the short follow-up period that may not have allowed the pulp to clear the SDF out through normal circulation [10]. In the same study, one tooth demonstrated the formation of tertiary dentin after 30 days of direct application of SDF on dental pulp. This finding was credited to the host immune response.

The SDF solution can swiftly penetrate dentin. A concern arises regarding the potential cytotoxic effects on the dentin-pulp complex due to the abundance of reactive ions in SDF. Studies have shown that reactive ions, such as silver ions, can permeate dentin to a depth ranging from 5 to 40 μm [11]. Some studies have also detected penetration of silver precipitates deeper than 2 mm in artificially demineralized dentin [12] and primary teeth [13]. In another study by Shijia Hu et al., it was demonstrated that the application of 38% SDF in teeth with a remaining dentin thickness of less than 1.0 mm, SDF was capable of causing the death of viable dental pulp stem cells [14]. A more recent study evaluated pulp cell response to SDF and potassium iodide and concluded that SDF applied alone caused cytotoxic effects on dental pulp, but a combination of SDF+ KI reduced the cytotoxic effects [15].

Studies have indicated that the toxic effects of silver and fluoride ions include depletion of glutathione and elevated oxidative stress or lipid peroxidation [16]. These processes diminish the antioxidant capabilities within the dental pulp, ultimately leading to cellular death and inflammation. Furthermore, research has demonstrated that the cytotoxic impact persists even after rinsing hydroxyapatite discs treated with SDF for 77 days [17]. In response, a proposed solution involves the application of glutathione alongside SDF to bolster antioxidant functions and mitigate the toxic effects exerted by SDF on dental pulp cells [16].

It has been studied that different chemical forms of silver may affect the viability of pulp cells to varying levels. Also, the nature of remaining dentin could affect the level of penetration of SDF. The remaining carious dentin could potentially be comprised of less tubular dentin or translucent dentin, or could even be partially or completely obstructed with sclerotic dentin [18].

#### *4.1.2 Tertiary dentin formation*

Tertiary dentin can be categorized as either reactionary or reparative in nature. Reactionary dentin is produced by existing odontoblasts, whereas reparative dentin is synthesized by newly differentiated odontoblast-like cells. Numerous factors influence the formation of tertiary dentin, including the method of cavity preparation, the condition of the dentin–restoration interface, the presence of bacteria, the type and application technique of the restorative material employed, and the amount and nature of remaining dentin thickness, among others.

An in-vivo comparative study by Korwar et al., conducted histological analysis, showcasing the deposition of tertiary dentin within the space between the pulp and the remaining dentin thickness [4], suggesting that SDF can be effectively used as an indirect pulp therapeutic agent. In a study conducted by Gotjamanos, silver fluoride displayed a positive pulp response, marked by the presence of ample reparative dentin and a broad odontoblastic layer [19].

Following SDF application, dentin remineralization is facilitated, resulting in the formation of an outer layer of highly mineralized dentin measuring approximately 150 μ. This layer exhibits a notable presence of calcium and phosphate ions [20] As a result of this remineralization process, dentin carious lesions treated with 38% SDF demonstrate increased microhardness. Microhardness serves as an indirect measure, or surrogate outcome, to gauge alterations in the mineral content of mineralized tissue. This effect was demonstrated in an ex vivo study involving primary upper anterior teeth with dentin carious lesions, which received 38% SDF treatment (administered once every 12 months) [21].

In a recent case report and review of literature, D. Mudumba illuminated a compelling instance of reparative dentin formation observed in a primary molar. This phenomenon effectively obviated the necessity for a more extensive pulp therapy procedure [22].

### 4.2 Indirect effects

#### *4.2.1 Pulp cell activity after indirect application*

The indirect application of SDF has been shown to increase the activity of pulpal cells adjacent to the carious lesion. It was also observed that the odontoblasts within the pulp close to the area of SDF application retained their flattened appearance [23]. This shape of odontoblasts might indicate their status after forming tertiary dentin3 [24]. Another indication of change in odontoblastic activity after SDF application is the presence of the Line of Owen that marks changes in cellular activity [4].

#### *4.2.2 Antimicrobial activity*

Oral flora is comprised of numerous species of bacteria, but *Streptococcus*, *Lactobacillus*, and *Actinomyces naeslundi* have been found to be associated with dentin and root caries [25]. The antimicrobial nature of SDF can be attributed to silver and fluoride ions. Silver ions are well-known for their broad-spectrum antimicrobial properties. They have the ability to disrupt multiple cellular processes in microorganisms, including bacterial cell wall synthesis, DNA replication, protein function, and enzymatic activity. Upon application, silver ions released from SDF penetrate the bacterial cell membrane, leading to structural damage and cell death [26]. Silver ions can also inhibit bacterial adhesion and biofilm formation on tooth surfaces, thereby reducing the colonization and growth of cariogenic bacteria like *Streptococcus mutans* and *Lactobacillus* species. Additionally, in a recent investigation by Sulyanto et al. (**Figure 1**) examining the impact of SDF on microbial communities within subsurface dentin with the help of 16S rRNA gene amplification and sequencing, it was found

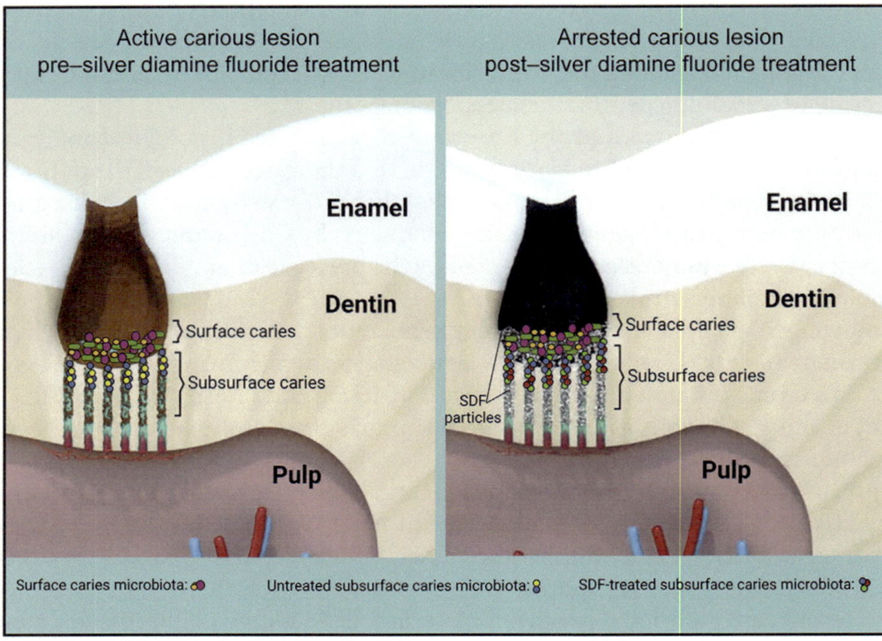


**Figure 1.**
*The impact of silver diamine fluoride (SDF) treatment on the microbial population within dentin structures.*

that SDF did not have much effect on microbial population on dentin surface but definitely altered the microbial composition deep within the dentin tubules [27].

Silver ions exhibit high reactivity and have a strong affinity for thiol groups (SH), which are prevalent in enzymes. When silver ions bind to these thiol groups, they denature the enzymes, rendering them non-functional. Consequently, the organism's energy system is disrupted, leading to the inability to maintain osmotic pressure. This disruption ultimately results in leakage of vital substrates, leading to cellular death [28].

The reaction of SDF with the thiol groups is based on the following equation:

$$A / N - SH + AgX \rightarrow A / N - S - AgX + HX \qquad (1)$$

(A/N is amino or nucleic acid; SH is the thiol group; Ag is silver; and X is diamine fluoride).

SDF inhibits the formation of biofilm and caries progression by killing bacteria [29]. SDF is effective against *Streptococcus mutans* and also *Actinomyces*, *Lactobacilli*, and other species [30]. Silver particles observed on the dentin surface following SDF treatment in vitro have been correlated with reduced bacterial counts and an increased presence of deceased bacteria [30]. Further in vitro investigations have demonstrated that SDF exhibits superior efficacy against *Streptococcus mutans* compared to silver nitrate or sodium fluoride alone. This suggests the combined contributions of both the silver and fluoride components of SDF to its potent antibacterial activity [30]. Alongside its cariostatic properties, the application of 38% SDF creates an environment that hinders the activation of dentin collagen enzymes [31].

Dentine surfaces treated with SDF exhibited significantly lower growth of *Streptococcus mutans* compared to untreated surfaces [32]. It was also demonstrated in another study that the colony-forming unit (CFU) counts of monospecies strains of *Streptococcus mutans* and *Actinomyces naeslundii* were notably reduced following SDF application, with few viable bacteria remaining [3]. Furthermore, CFU counts of dual-species biofilms containing *Streptococcus mutans* and *Lactobacillus acidophilus* were markedly lower on demineralized dentine treated with SDF compared to those treated with water alone. Additionally, the dead-to-live ratios of bacteria were significantly higher after SDF application than after water application [33].

It was also noted in another study that the adhesiveness and growth of *Lactobacillus casei*, *Streptococcus mutans,* and *Streptococcus oralis* reduced after treating the surface with SDF [34].

#### *4.2.3 Dentin remineralization*

To understand the physiology of dentin remineralization, it is necessary to understand the following chemical reaction that takes place when SDF is applied to the tooth surface,

$$Ca_{10}\left(PO_4\right)_6\left(OH\right)_2 + Ag\left(NH_3\right)2\mathrm{F} \rightarrow CaF_2 + \mathrm{AgPO_4} + NH_4OH \qquad (2)$$

(hydroxyapatite+ silver diamine fluoride →calcium fluoride+ silver phosphate+ ammonium hydroxide)

Later, calcium fluoride dissociates into calcium and fluoride, leading to the formation of insoluble fluorapatite. The calcium fluoride formed after the application of SDF functions like a pH-regulated fluoride reservoir on the tooth surface [35]. It is important to note here that 38% of SDF contains 44,800 ppm fluoride, which is probably the highest among the fluoride agents in dentistry. This fluoride promotes the remineralization of carious dentin.

Also, silver phosphate is unstable and highly soluble and gets reduced back into silver ions that may react with the readily available chloride ions to form lower-soluble silver chloride ($AgCl_2$). The deposition of silver chloride causes the black appearance of tooth surface after the application of SDF [36]. The silver ions also react with the collagen in the dentin and get reduced to metallic silver. The more demineralized the dentin is, the more collagen is exposed and available to react with silver ions, thus resulting in more metallic silver formation. This process results in black discoloration [37].

#### *4.2.4 Reduction in dentin hypersensitivity*

There is still no consensus on the exact mechanism of dentin hypersensitivity, but Brannstrom's hydrodynamic theory is the most plausible hypothesis. It states that any thermal, chemical, or mechanical stimuli can alter the direction or flow of dentinal tubular fluid, which in turn stimulates the A-delta fibers surrounding the odontoblasts.

SDF was cleared by The United States Food and Drug Administration in 2014 to treat dentine hypersensitivity. One proposed mechanism of action of SDF is the formation of a squamous layer formed by the aqueous solutions of silver and fluoride over the exposed dentin and that seals the dentinal tubules, thus reducing the fluid shift in the tubules that is responsible for sensitivity [10]. Another hypothesis is the formation of calcium fluoride by the interaction of fluoride ions and free calcium ions that block the dentinal tubules [38]. This calcium fluoride is partially soluble in saliva [39]. Scanning electron microscopic studies of SDF-treated dentin have revealed the presence of silver particles within the tubules, thereby decreasing their diameter and eventually decreasing the tubular fluid movement [40].

A systematic review by Piovesan et al. in 2023 concluded that 38% SDF is beneficial in treating dentin hypersensitivity, but longer evaluation periods are required to assess its efficacy in the long term [41]. Not much consistency has been seen in various studies testing the effect of SDF in reducing dentin hypersensitivity.

Castillo JL studied the clinical effectiveness of topical SDF as a desensitizing agent and concluded SDF to be safe and efficient in treating dentin hypersensitivity after 24 h and 7 days [42]. Another study analyzed the efficacy of SDF and $CO_2$ laser in dentin hypersensitivity and found a reduction in visual analog scale (VAS) and DIAGNOdent scores after the application of SDF alone or along with Co2 laser [43]. A more recent study evaluated the effectiveness of 38% SDF in reducing dentine hypersensitivity in exposed root surfaces in older Chinese adults. This study concluded that 38% SDF was more effective than 5% potassium nitrate solution in reducing hypersensitivity on exposed root surfaces [44].

## 5. Adverse effects of SDF

The most common adverse effects of the application of SDF are pulpal irritation, staining, and soft tissue irritation [29]. It has been studied that tooth staining can be reduced by the application of potassium iodide immediately after SDF [32].

Pulpal irritation is found to be more pronounced in deep cavities where the remaining dentin thickness is less than 1.0 mm [14]. Temporary staining on skin or submucosa resolves within 2 weeks by natural exfoliation [45].

In the event of accidental ingestion of a large volume of SDF, a 10% calcium gluconate solution can be administered to facilitate the formation of insoluble calcium fluoride that will eventually be eliminated from the body [45].

## 6. International guidelines

The American Academy of Pediatric Dentistry's policy statement (2023) supports the use of SDF as a minimally invasive caries management option to prevent or delay the need for more extensive procedures and promotes the appropriate training and education to dental personnel in accordance with the respective state's dental practice act. It also encourages further practice-based research aimed at evaluating the efficacy and impact of SDF on the health-related quality of life of infants, children, adolescents, and individuals with special healthcare needs [46].

## 7. Conclusion

In conclusion, SDF emerges as a valuable tool in contemporary dentistry, offering multifaceted benefits for caries management, dentin hypersensitivity relief, and preventive care. Its non-invasive nature, cost-effectiveness, and ease of application make it particularly well-suited for addressing the diverse needs of various patient populations, including children, older adults, and individuals with special healthcare needs. Moreover, amidst the challenges posed by the COVID-19 pandemic, SDF stands out as a safe and compliant alternative that aligns with public health guidelines. However, further research and practice-based studies are warranted to fully elucidate its long-term efficacy and impact on oral health-related quality of life across different demographics. Overall, SDF represents a promising advancement in modern dental practice, poised to enhance preventive care strategies and improve oral health outcomes for patients worldwide.

## Conflict of interest

The authors declare no conflict of interest.

## Author details

Divya Mudumba
SmileWorks Family Dentistry, Pittsfield, Massachusetts, USA

*Address all correspondence to: mdivya.dmd@gmail.com

## References

[1] Yamaga R, Nishino M, Yoshida S, et al. Diamine silver fluoride and its clinical application. The Journal of Osaka University Dental School. 1972;**12**:1-20

[2] Fung MH. Arresting early childhood caries with silver diamine fluoride: A literature review. Journal of Oral Hygiene & Health. 2013;**01**(03):1-5. DOI: 10.4172/2332-0702.1000117

[3] Chu CH, Mei L, Seneviratne CJ, Lo ECM. Effects of silver diamine fluoride on dentine carious lesions induced by *Streptococcus* mutans and *Actinomyces naeslundii* biofilms. International Journal of Paediatric Dentistry. 2012;**22**(1):2-10

[4] Korwar A, Sharma S, Logani A, Shah N. Pulp response to high fluoride releasing glass ionomer, silver diamine fluoride, and calcium hydroxide used for indirect pulp treatment: An invivo comparative study. Contemporary Clinical Dentistry. 2015;**6**(3):288-292

[5] Gregory D, Hyde S. Root caries in older adults. Journal of the California Dental Association. 2015;**43**:439-445

[6] Crystal YO, Marghalani AA, Ureles SD, Wright JT, Sulyanto R, Divaris K, et al. Use of silver diamine fluoride for dental caries management in children and adolescents, including those with special health care needs. Pediatric Dentistry. 2017;**39**(5):135-145

[7] Raskin SE, Tranby EP, Ludwig S, Okunev I, Frantsve-Hawley J, Boynes S. Survival of silver diamine fluoride among patients treated in community dental clinics: A naturalistic study. BMC Oral Health. 2021;**21**(1):35. DOI: 10.1186/s12903-020-01379-x

[8] Wright T, Slade G, Meyer B, Lampiris L, et al. Non-surgical caries management approaches: Treatment recommendations during the COVID_19 pandemic. Available from: https://oralhealthnc.org/primary_resources/non-surgical-caries-management-approaches/

[9] Bagher SM, Sabbagh HJ, AlJohani SM, et al. Parental acceptance of the utilization of silver diamine fluoride on their child's primary and permanent teeth. Patient Preference and Adherence. 2019;**23**(13):829-835

[10] Greenwall-Cohen J, Greenwall L, Barry S. Silver diamine fluoride - an overview of the literature and current clinical techniques. British Dental Journal. 2020;**228**(11):831-838. DOI: 10.1038/s41415-020-1641-4

[11] Willershausen I, Schulte D, Azaripour A, Weyer V, Briseno B, Willershausen B. Penetration potential of a silver diamine fluoride solution on dentin surfaces. An ex vivo study. Clinical Laboratory. 2015;**61**:1695-1701

[12] Jiang RD, Lin H, Zheng G, Zhang XM, Du Q, Yang M. In vitro dentin barrier cytotoxicity testing of some dental restorative materials. Journal of Dentistry. 2017;**58**:28-33

[13] Xie H, Chua M, Islam I, Bentini R, Cao T, Viana-Gomes JC, et al. CVD-grown monolayer graphene induces osteogenic but not odontoblastic differentiation of dental pulp stem cells. Dental Materials. 2017;**33**(1):e13-e21

[14] Shijia T et al. Characterization of silver diamine fluoride cytotoxicity

using microfluidic tooth-on-a-chip and gingival equivalents. Dental Materials. 2022;**38**(8):1385-1394

[15] Fernandes LO, Mendes Soares IP, Anselmi C, Pires MLBA, Ribeiro RAO, Peruchi V, et al. Pulp cell response to the application of silver diamine fluoride and potassium iodide on caries-like demineralized dentin. Clinical Oral Investigations. 2023;**27**(12):7295-7306. DOI: 10.1007/s00784-023-05320-8

[16] Kim S, Nassar M, Tamura Y, Hiraishi N, Jamleh A, Nikaido T, et al. The effect of reduced glutathione on the toxicity of silver diamine fluoride in rat pulpal cells. Journal of Applied Oral Science. 2021;**29**:e20200859

[17] Fancher ME, Fournier S, Townsend J, Lallier TE. Cytotoxic effects of silver diamine fluoride. American Journal of Dentistry. 2019;**32**:152-156

[18] Manuschai J et al. Penetration of silver diamine fluoride in deep carious lesions of human permanent teeth: An In vitro study. International Journal of Dentistry. 2021;**2021**:3059129

[19] Gotjamanos T. Pulp response in primary teeth with deep residual caries treated with silver fluoride and glass ionomer cement ('atraumatic' technique). Australian Dental Journal. 1996;**41**:328-334

[20] Mei ML, Ito L, Cao Y, Lo EC, Li Q, Chu C. An ex vivo study of arrested primary teeth caries with silver diamine fluoride therapy. Journal of Dentistry. 2014;**42**:395-402

[21] Chu CH, Lo EC. Microhardness of dentine in primary teeth after topical fluoride applications. Journal of Dentistry. 2008;**36**:387-391. DOI: 10.1016/j.jdent.2008.02.013

[22] Mudumba D et al. Reparative dentin formation by silver diamine fluoride- a case report and review of literature. Journal of the Massachusetts Dental Society. 2023;**72**(3):24-25

[23] Bimstein E, Damm D. Human primary tooth histology six months after treatment with silver diamine fluoride. The Journal of Clinical Pediatric Dentistry. 2018;**42**(6):442-444

[24] Tashiro Y, Itota T, Takagi R, Shinno Y, Yoshiyama M. Distribution of calbindin D-28k in odontoblasts after cavity preparation in human teeth. Journal of Oral Tissue Engineering. 2005;**3**(1):1-6

[25] Hahn C-L, Falkler WA, Minah GE. Microbiological studies of carious dentine from human teeth with irreversible pulpitis. Archives of Oral Biology. 1991;**36**(2):147-153

[26] Coward JE, Carr HS, Rosenkranz HS. Silver sulfadiazine: Effect on the ultrastructure of *Pseudomonas aeruginosa*. Antimicrobial Agents and Chemotherapy. 1973;**3**(5):621-624

[27] Sulyanto T et al. Silver diamine fluoride alters microbial communities in subsurface dentin. JADA Foundational Science. 2022;**1**:100004

[28] Bragg PD, Rainnie DJ. The effect of silver ions on the respiratory chain of Escherichia coli. Canadian Journal of Microbiology. 1974;**20**(6):883-889

[29] Rosenblatt A, Stamford TCM, Niederman R. Silver diamine fluoride: a caries "silver-fluoride bullet". Journal of Dental Research. 2009;**88**(2):116-125

[30] Zhao IS, Gao SS, Hiraishi N, et al. Mechanisms of silver diamine fluoride on arresting caries: A literature

review. International Dental Journal. 2018;**68**(2):67-76. DOI: 10.1111/idj.12320

[31] Mei M, Lo E, Chu C. Arresting dentine caries with silver diamine fluoride: What's behind it? Journal of Dental Research. 2018;**97**:751-758

[32] Knight G, McIntyre J, Craig G, et al. An in vitro model to measure the effect of a silver fluoride and potassium iodide treatment on the permeability of demineralized dentine to *Streptococcus mutans*. Australian Dental Journal. 2005;**50**:242-245

[33] Mei ML, Chu CH, Low KH, et al. Caries arresting effect of silver diamine fluoride on dentine carious lesion with *S. mutans* and *L. acidophilus* dual-species cariogenic biofilm. Medicina Oral, Patología Oral y Cirugía Bucal. 2013;**18**:824-831

[34] de Almeida LF, Cavalcanti YW, Valenca A. In vitro antibacterial activity of silver diamine fluoride in different concentrations. Acta Odontológica Latinoamericana. 2011;**24**:127-131

[35] Mei ML, Nudelman F, Marzec B, Walker JM, Lo ECM, Walls AW, et al. Formation of fluorohydroxyapatite with silver diamine fluoride. Journal of Dental Research. 2017;**96**:1122-1128

[36] Li Y, Qiu X, Li J, et al. Effect of a silver ammonia fluoride solution on the prevention and inhibition of caries. Zhonghua Kou Qiang Ke Za Zhi. 1984;**19**:97-100

[37] Sayed M, Matsui N, Uo M, Nikaido T, Oikawa M, Burrow MF, et al. Morphological and elemental analysis of silver penetration into sound/demineralized dentin after SDF application. Dental Materials. 2019;**35**(12)

[38] Orchardson R, Gilliam D. Managing dentin hypersensitivity. Journal of the American Dental Association (1939). 2006;**137**:990-998

[39] Craig GG, Knight GM, Mcintyre JM. Clinical evaluation of diamine silver fluoride/potassium iodide as a dentine desensitizing agent. A pilot study. Australian Dental Journal. 2012;**57**(3):308-311

[40] Li Y, Liu Y, Psoter WJ, Nguyen OM, Bromage TG, Walters MA, et al. Assessment of the silver penetration and distribution in carious lesions of deciduous teeth treated with silver diamine fluoride. Caries Research. 2019;**53**(4):431-440

[41] Piovesan ÉTA, Alves JB, Ribeiro CDPV, Massignan C, Bezerra ACB, Leal SC. Is silver diamine fluoride effective in reducing dentin hypersensitivity? A systematic review. Journal of Dental Research, Dental Clinics, Dental Prospects. 2023;**17**(2):63-70. DOI: 10.34172/joddd.2023.35449

[42] Castillo J, Rivera S, Aparicio T, et al. The short-term effects of diamine silver fluoride on tooth sensitivity: A randomized controlled trial. Journal of Dental Research. 2011;**90**(2):203-208

[43] Permata N, Rahardjo A, Adiatman M, Samnieng P. Efficacy of silver diamine fluoride and combination with $CO_2$ laser in reducing dentin hypersensitivity. Journal of Physics Conference Series. 2018;**1073**(6):62001

[44] Chan AKY, Tsang YC, Jiang CM, Leung KCM, Lo ECM, Chu CH. Treating hypersensitivity in older adults with silver diamine fluoride. A randomised clinical trial. Journal of Dental. 2023;**136**:104616

[45] Wu MY, Suryanarayanan K, van Ooij WJ, Oerther DB. Using microbial genomics to evaluate the effectiveness of silver to prevent biofilm formation. Water Science and Technology. 2007;**55**(8-9):413-419

[46] American Academy of Pediatric Dentistry. Policy on the use of silver diamine fluoride for pediatric dental patients. In: The Reference Manual of Pediatric Dentistry. Chicago, IL: American Academy of Pediatric Dentistry; 2023. pp. 103-105

Chapter 7

# Biomaterials for Regeneration of the Dentin-Pulp Complex

*Cristian Danilo Urgiles Urgiles,*
*Cristina Estefania Urgiles Esquivel,*
*Maria Isabel Bravo, Fernanda Gonzalez*
*and Daniela San Martin*

## Abstract

Biomaterials or bioactive materials interact with the surrounding environment, stimulating growth and promoting the regeneration of damaged or lost dental tissues. They can be natural, derived from animal or plant tissues, synthetic like bioceramics, or a combination of both. Natural biomaterials include substances from animal or plant tissues like dentin, bone, and collagen, while synthetic ones include materials like bioceramics, bioactive glass, and polymers. These materials are used in various dental treatments such as direct pulp capping, indirect pulp capping, partial and total pulpotomy, and pulp regeneration. This method aims to promote pulp healing and the formation of a mineralized tissue barrier, avoiding more invasive and extensive treatments. The formation of mineralized tissue is considered a favorable response of the exposed pulp tissue, showing its ability to recover. Different biomaterials, their mechanisms of action, clinical indications, applications, and future perspectives will be described in this chapter.

**Keywords:** biomaterials, regeneration, dentin-pulp complex, pulp tissue, dentin

## 1. Introduction

Regenerative dentistry represents a paradigm as it aims to reconstruct dental tissues using the potential of stem cells and bioactive materials [1]. Stem cells possess the ability to differentiate, repair, and regulate inflammation. Bei Li et al. have demonstrated that stem cells also exhibit clonogenic capacity and the ability to differentiate into various stromal lineages [2]. Bioactive materials like calcium phosphate (CaP) and silicate-based materials interact with the surrounding environment, stimulating biocompatibility and the capacity to induce cell migration, proliferation, and differentiation. Among the biomaterials available are collagen hydrogels that promote cell adhesion and differentiation [1]. Ceramic biomaterials such as hydroxyapatite and tricalcium phosphate have been shown to stimulate dentin formation and support tissue repair [3]. Synthetic and natural biomaterials, including autologous, allogeneic, and xenogeneic materials, as well as nanostructured or microporous biomaterials composed of hydroxyapatite nanoparticles in three dimensions [4, 5].

In this context, the selection and evaluation of biomaterials play a crucial role in the success of these procedures. This chapter aims to thoroughly explore the range of biomaterials, their mechanisms of action in dentin-pulp regeneration analyzing their long-term efficacy, interaction with surrounding tissues, and applicability in clinical settings. Existing clinical studies will be critically examined to provide a comprehensive overview of current advancements and suggest potential directions for future research to enhance treatment personalization and address ethical and safety challenges.

## 2. Biomaterials used in regeneration of the dentin-pulp complex

Biomaterials play an integral role in the dentin-pulp regeneration process by providing both physical and biological support. They are classified based on various criteria (e.g., **Table 1**).

To achieve the safest tissue response and optimize outcomes in therapies, new complex biomaterials have emerged to preserve pulp vitality during conservative operations and restorative dental procedures [9, 12]. However, the wide range of biomaterials available for dentin-pulp coating (DPC) should possess several characteristics, including ease of manipulation during operative procedures, adhesion to dental substrate, antibacterial properties, excellent sealing ability, insolubility in tissue fluids, biocompatibility, bioactivity, radiopacity, absence of tooth discoloration, and

| | | | |
|---|---|---|---|
| Composition | • Natural biomaterials: | Derived from natural sources such as dentin, enamel, collagen, or stem cells. | |
| | • Synthetic biomaterials: | Manufactured using synthetic materials like cements, resins, or polymers. | |
| | • Hybrid biomaterials: | Combine natural and synthetic materials [4]. | |
| Mechanism of action | • Bioactive biomaterials: | These biomaterials interact with pulp tissue to stimulate the formation of new tissue. | |
| | • Biomimetic biomaterials: | These biomaterials imitate the structure and function of natural tissues. | |
| | • Combined biomaterials: | These biomaterials combine two or more types to achieve a synergistic effect [4]. | |
| Function | • Coating biomaterials: | These biomaterials are used to protect dental pulp from infection and irritation. | Biodentine [6].<br>MTA [7].<br>Bioactive Glass [8]. |
| | • Matrix biomaterials for new tissue formation: | These biomaterials provide physical support for the formation of new tissue. | Collagen Biomaterials [3].<br>Hydroxyapatite Biomaterials [9].<br>Polymer Biomaterials [10]. |
| | • Growth factor-releasing biomaterials: | These biomaterials release growth factors that stimulate the formation of new tissue [4]. | Biomaterials with cell adhesion proteins [10, 11].<br>Biomaterials with isolated growth factors [10, 11].<br>Biomaterials with complex growth factors [10, 11]. |

**Table 1.**
*Classification of biomaterials for dentin-pulp regeneration according different criteria.*

promotion of mineralized tissue barrier formation. Unfortunately, no current DPC biomaterial possesses all these characteristics [13].

### 2.1 Calcium hydroxide (CH)

Calcium hydroxide is a chemical compound with the formula Ca(OH)2 and a basic pH of 12.5–13.5 due to the release of hydroxyl ions, which helps protect the pulp tissue by stimulating fibroblasts [14]. For decades, it has been considered a standard material for DPC, possessing antimicrobial activity and the ability to remineralizer carious dentin [15–17].

Disadvantage: Its main drawback is inadequate adhesion to hard tissues, failing to provide optimal sealing.

Another disadvantage of calcium hydroxide is its capacity to dissolve. However, the specific mechanism responsible for dissolution in the tissue remains largely unexplored in the existing literature and requires further research [18, 19].

*Mechanism of action:*

It leads to a tunnel-like phenomenon in the dentin bridge, although this imperfection decreases as the dentin bridge thickness increases [15, 20].

When placed over exposed pulp, it shows satisfactory clinical outcomes as a material for DPC in superficial necrosis [14], stimulating the formation of a reparative dentin bridge through cellular differentiation, extracellular matrix secretion, and potential mineralization, creating a microenvironment oversaturated with calcium ions in close proximity to the pulp. The effectiveness of calcium hydroxide depends on the application type and the severity of the pulp injury; it is effective in protecting the pulp from infection and inflammation but is not always effective in regenerating it. Long-term clinical research on DPC follow-up using calcium hydroxide has yielded success rates ranging from 37% to 81.8%. This observation remains consistent despite multiple studies demonstrating the effectiveness of calcium hydroxide in promoting pulp healing [14, 21]. Findings from studies with follow-up durations exceeding 5 years have shown a broad success rate: 77.6% between 2 and 6 years, 58.7% up to 9 years, and over 10 years, 72.7% [22].

*Clinical applications:*

- Direct Pulp Capping: Calcium hydroxide is applied directly to the exposed dental pulp to create a physical barrier that protects the pulp tissue.
- Regenerative Pulp Therapy involves the use of CH as a base as it has the ability to restore dental pulp through the process of differentiation, leading to the formation of odontoblasts, dentin, and blood vessels [9, 20].
- Deep Caries: Remineralizes carious dentin and prevents pulp exposure.
- Irreversible Pulp Lesions: It can be used to relieve pain and inflammation in cases [9, 20].

*Contraindications:*

- Should not be used in cases of active pulpal infection.
- Apical root fracture.

*Side effects:*

- Common and transient side effects of calcium hydroxide include: burning sensation, sensitivity to touch, slight inflammation in the treated area for a few days [9, 20].

## 2.2 Bioceramic cements

### *2.2.1 Mineral trioxide aggregate (MTA)*

It is a biomaterial derived from Portland cement, its main components consist of tricalcium silicate, dicalcium silicate, and tricalcium aluminate, supplemented with bismuth oxide to improve radiopacity [23]. Initially developed for apical perforation repair procedures, it is currently a versatile material with bioactive properties that have expanded its use to regenerative dentistry due to its ability to form a dentin barrier, stimulate the formation of hard tissues, and exhibit low cellular toxicity [24–26]. This material presents the following beneficial properties for pulp repair:

- Exceptional biocompatibility when applied to the pulp wound
- Sealing capacity that facilitates excellent cell/material adhesion
- Low solubility
- Prevents bacterial infiltration
- Stimulation of mineralized matrix formation [24].

*Mechanism of action:*

It exhibits physicochemical properties due to the release of calcium ions and the alkalinity of the material, inducing the formation of reparative dentin by attracting and activating cells responsible for the formation of hard tissues, thus contributing to the development of a matrix and the mineralization process [27, 28].

It triggers the migration of progenitor cells (specifically fibroblasts) from the central pulp to the site of exposure. This process helps improve their replication and specialization into odontoblast-like cells while avoiding the induction of apoptosis in pulp cells [27].

MTA initiates a time-dependent pro-inflammatory environment that facilitates wound regeneration through positive regulation of cytokines. Positive regulation of cytokines is responsible for stimulating biomineralization, achieved by the production of collagen fibrils or apatite-like groups at the interface between dentin and MTA. The release of calcium ions by MTA induces antibacterial effects and promotes mineralization in the area beneath the exposed pulp, potentially preserving pulp vitality. When used in conjunction with a sealed restoration, MTA prevents bacterial leakage and may help preserve pulp tissue, facilitate healing, and maintain pulp vitality [29, 30]. The primary calcium ion released by MTA participates in a reaction with phosphates present in tissue fluid, resulting in hydroxyapatite formation. This process makes the material biocompatible and capable of ensuring sufficient sealing [31, 32].

*Advantages:*

The inflammatory response triggered by MTA is transient and less severe compared to that induced by CH [33].

It has the ability to decrease levels of inflammation, hyperemia, and pulpal necrosis, while also being able to dissolve the bioactive proteins involved in the tooth repair process [28].

*Disadvantages:*

Extended setting time, which can be several hours.

Difficult material manipulation.

Discoloration, currently countered with new presentations (MTA WHITE).

High cost [17, 26, 34].

*Clinical application of MTA in pulp-dentin regeneration:*

*Pulpotomy and partial pulpotomy*

Apexification and periapical Surgery: Used to promote apical formation and closure in cases of open apices or periapical lesions.

Retroapical filling and endodontic surgery: Preferred material for retrograde filling in endodontic surgery [35].

Direct pulp capping in situations of pulp exposure, for its ability to promote reactive dentin formation [36].

*Efficiency*

Efficiency in apexification, with positive results in root apex regeneration [37]. Recent research studies have presented findings indicating that MTA demonstrates a higher rate of clinical success, induces a lower degree of pulpal inflammatory response, and facilitates the formation of mineralized tissue barriers compared to CH in DPC [38–40]. A comprehensive study involving 49 teeth with carious pulp exposure in 37 patients, where MTA was used, revealed an overall success rate of 97.96% after a span of 9 years [31]. The authors of this study claimed that MTA, when used in a two-visit treatment protocol, shows potential as a pulp capping material for direct exposures in permanent teeth [31]. In another study covering 122 teeth with caries and mechanical exposure in 108 patients, both MTA and CH were used for capping. The overall success rate of MTA for carious and mechanical exposure was 80% and 70%, respectively, while for CH it was 62% and 50%, respectively, after a duration of 1 to 6.6 years. The study concluded that after DPC, MTA appears to be more effective than CH in maintaining long-term pulpal vitality [41].

A recent study conducted on 229 teeth with mechanical and carious exposure in 205 patients, using MTA and CH, revealed an overall success rate of 80% and 84% for MTA in cases of mechanical and carious exposure, respectively, while for CH, it was 57% and 70%, respectively, after a duration of 2 to 10 and 25 year. The findings of this study suggested that when used as a DPC agent, MTA provides better long-term results compared to CH, and immediate placement of a permanent restoration after DPC was recommended. Within the parameters of these studies, MTA appears to be a suitable substitute for CH in DPC [11]. Therefore, it can be stated that MTA has been established as a suitable protective agent and a reliable treatment option for exposed pulp, with a certain degree of predictability in DPC [5].

### *2.2.2 Biodentine – dentin substitute*

Biodentine, a biomaterial developed by Septodont in Saint-Maur-des-Fossés, France [26], has emerged as a prominent choice for dentin-pulp complex regeneration. It is a mixture of powder and liquid components containing tricalcium silicate, tricalcium aluminate, calcium carbonate, and water, demonstrating notable bioactive characteristics by releasing calcium and silicate ions [41]. Unlike other materials, it does not contain inorganic compounds such as calcium aluminate, calcium sulfate, or bismuth oxide [26, 42].

The documented efficacy of Biodentine in the dentin-pulp complex for mechanically exposed pulps is comparable to that of MTA [32].

*Advantages:*

- It has better mechanical properties.
- Improved color stability.
- Simpler application process.
- Faster initial setting time compared to MTA [4, 39, 43–45].

*Disadvantages:*

- It has limitations in terms of radiopacity and achieving the desired or optimized consistency.
- Controlled release and regeneration of ions with Biodentine may not meet all clinical needs.

Despite its limitations, Biodentine remains a valuable option in dentistry for a variety of procedures, thanks to its bioactive properties and its ability to promote dentin-pulp tissue regeneration.

Controlled release of ions by Biodentine promotes mineralization and hard tissue formation, favoring dentin-pulp regeneration, emphasizing Biodentine's ability to induce reparative dentin formation and its excellent biocompatibility. Biodentine has been found to release significantly higher amounts of calcium compared to CH cement and MTA [46–49]. An increase in the amount of released calcium indicates a simultaneous increase in hydroxyl ions. The antibacterial properties of Biodentine are attributed to its high pH, achieved through the action of hydroxyl ions on the surrounding tissue [19]. Due to the elevated pH, a thin layer of coagulative necrosis forms between the vital pulp tissue and the pulp capping material [50]. This necrotic zone acts as a barrier between the alkaline substance pH and the pulp cells beneath it. Additionally, a reparative dentin bridge will form adjacent to it. Furthermore, Biodentine has been observed to release silicon ions into the surrounding dentin. It is hypothesized that these silicon ions produced by Biodentine aid in the formation of dentin bridges and accelerate mineralization [42]. Studies have shown that after applying Biodentine for DPC, a complete dentin bridge forms, accompanied by a less inflammatory pulpal response and well-arranged layers of odontoblasts and odontoblast-like cells [51].

*Clinical application of biodentine in dentin-pulp regeneration*

The clinical application of Biodentine in dentin and pulp restoration has been extensively studied. Research has compared the efficacy of Biodentine as a direct DPC material with that of MTA. In a 6-month evaluation, 24 teeth with carious pulp exposure were treated with MTA or Biodentine, resulting in overall success rates of

91.7% and 83.3%, respectively. Another experiment involving 68 teeth with carious pulp exposure in 54 patients showed that after 6 months of treatment, both MTA and Biodentine exhibited overall success rates of 93.5% and 93.1%, respectively. After a duration of 12 months, the achievement rates of MTA and Biodentine were 100% and 96%, respectively. A subsequent 3-year study revealed overall success rates for MTA and Biodentine of 96% and 91.7%, respectively. These findings imply that when used as materials for dental pulp coverage in fully mature permanent teeth with carious exposure, both Biodentine and MTA demonstrate favorable and comparable success rates. However, the long-term achievement of dental pulp coverage may depend on the amount of remaining healthy dental structure and the resistance of the coronal restoration [52]. Nevertheless, further evidence from clinical trials with extended follow-up periods is needed to thoroughly evaluate the effectiveness of Biodentine in covering exposed dental pulp.

Pulpotomy and partial pulpotomy: Biodentine has been shown to be effective in pulpotomies, where it is applied in the pulp chamber to preserve the vitality of the affected pulp tissue. Significant success rates have been demonstrated in pulpotomies with Biodentine, with reparative dentin formation and a favorable pulpal response.

Direct pulpal sealing: In cases of direct pulp exposure during cavity preparations, Biodentine has been used for direct pulpal sealing. Its sealing capacity and compatibility with pulp tissues have been noted [6, 26].

Direct pulpal capping: In situations of indirect pulp exposure, Biodentine has been applied as a direct pulp capping material, yielding positive pulpal responses and reactive dentin formation when used as a direct capping agent [26].

The efficacy and prognosis of this therapy depend on variables such as age, type of exposure, site of exposure, and degree of pulp exposure. It is worth noting that MTA has undergone more extensive evaluation as a direct pulp capping substance compared to Biodentine. Furthermore, prevailing research on Biodentine has involved a smaller number of participants compared to MTA research [42].

### *2.2.3 BioAggregate*

BioAggregate is a bioinductive tricalcium cement [48], composed of tricalcium silicate, dicalcium silicate, monobasic calcium phosphate, amorphous silica, and tantalum oxide acting as a radiopacifier [34, 53]. Accumulated evidence suggests that when used as an apical filling material, BioAggregate exhibits exceptional sealing capabilities and superior biocompatibility compared to MTA. Additionally, recent research has provided empirical evidence indicating that BioAggregate outperforms MTA in terms of its ability to promote odontoblastic differentiation and mineralization when employed as a pulp capping material [54].

*Composition and properties*

BioAggregate, an advanced iteration of MTA, lacks aluminum. Instead, it is primarily composed of tantalum oxide, which replaces bismuth oxide and calcium phosphate. The removal of aluminum from its chemical composition leads to a reduction in adverse effects on inflammatory cellular response [34]. However, the effects of BioAggregate on dental pulp tissues have not been thoroughly investigated.

*Indications*

BioAggregate is used for dentin-pulp complex regeneration in the following cases:

- Irreversible pulp lesions: BioAggregate can be used to alleviate pain and inflammation in cases of irreversible pulp lesions.

- Irreversible pulp lesions with pulp exposure: BioAggregate can be used to protect exposed dental pulp from infections and inflammation.

- Irreversible pulp lesions with pulp exposure and apical root fracture: BioAggregate can be used to restore dental pulp function in cases of irreversible pulp lesions with pulp exposure and apical root fracture [54].

*Efficacy*

The efficacy of BioAggregate in dentin-pulp complex regeneration has been evaluated in various clinical research studies. Overall, these studies have demonstrated that BioAggregate is effective in stimulating dental pulp regeneration in cases of irreversible pulp lesions. Recent findings have indicated that MTA has exhibited significantly higher levels of thicker hard tissue development compared to BioAggregate. However, BioAggregate also showed substantial and uniform hard tissue barrier formation. Further examination is required to determine if BioAggregate could function as a suitable substitute for pulp capping materials [54].

*2.2.4 Super MTA paste*

It is composed of Portland cement, with the addition of TBB (tributyl borane) as a polymerization initiator, eliminating the need for photopolymerization [13]. It provides biocompatibility as a pulp-capping material and is capable of inducing the formation of a uniform dentin bridge. It is composed of:

- Zinc oxide, which has antimicrobial and antifungal properties.

- Bismuth oxide, with radiopaque properties, making it visible on radiographs.

- Tricalcium silicate, with cementing and bioactive properties.

- Bismuth orthosilicate, with cementing and antifungal properties [13, 29].

*Properties:*

- Biocompatibility with human tissues.

- Bioactivity, stimulating the regeneration of the dental pulp complex.

- Biodegradability, naturally decomposing in the body.

- Mechanical strength: The paste exhibits high mechanical strength, suitable for use in stress-prone areas [29].

*Clinical indications:*

- Indirect pulp therapy: Used to seal the pulp chamber and protect the dental pulp from infections.

- Pulp Regenerative Therapy: Can be used as a base for applying dental pulp or periodontal ligament stem cells.

- Direct pulp capping: To protect exposed dental pulp from infections.
- Sealing an open apex of a tooth [27, 29, 55].

*Efficacy:*

Super MTA paste has demonstrated therapeutic efficacy comparable to TheraCal LC when applied to exposed pulp. However, further clinical trials are needed to validate its efficacy in both short- and long-term clinical outcomes [27, 55].

### 2.3 Resin-based MTA: TheraCal LC

*Composition and properties:*

TheraCal LC (Bisco, Schaumburg, IL, USA) [32], considered as a resin-based biomaterial, is composed of calcium silicate and can be used as a pulp-capping agent and as a protective lining combined with restoration materials [22]. Its composition includes type I collagen, hydroxyapatite, fibronectin, and growth factors. The collagen matrix provides a solid framework for dentin-pulp complex restoration. Hydroxyapatite acts as a supportive scaffold for dentin and blood vessel formation. Fibronectin helps facilitate cellular adhesion and migration, while growth factors serve as catalysts for the dentin-pulp complex regeneration process. In order to address the limitations of the original MTA, certain resin-modified MTAs have been introduced with the aim of reducing setting time [32].

TheraCal LC has effectively demonstrated its ability to release calcium ions, which are essential in stimulating and differentiating human dental pulp cells and odontoblasts, as well as aiding in the formation of new mineralized hard tissues [23, 47, 56].

*Applications:*

TheraCal LC is used in dentin-pulp complex regeneration in cases of irreversible pulp lesions and can be employed to protect exposed dental pulp from infections and inflammation [18, 47].

*Efficacy:*

The efficacy of TheraCal LC in stimulating dentin-pulp complex regeneration has been evaluated in various clinical research studies and has shown success in promoting dental pulp regeneration in cases of irreversible pulp lesions. Clinical success rates of TheraCal LC have been evaluated and compared with other substances over a short period of time [57]. It has been determined that there is no statistically significant difference in success rates among TheraCal, Biodentine, and MTA when compared with each other, leading to the recommendation of TheraCal LC as a substance for dentin-pulp complex restoration [32, 57].

### 2.4 Collagen hydrogels

Collagen hydrogels are biomaterials composed of a collagen matrix and a liquid substance. Collagen is a protein naturally found in the human body and possesses biocompatible, bioactive, and biodegradable properties. The liquid substance can be water, blood serum, or saline solution [58–61].

*Indications:*

Collagen hydrogels are used for various clinical indications in dentistry, including pulp regeneration, promoting regeneration in cases of irreversible lesions, closure of open apices, in regenerative pulp therapy as a base for the application of dental pulp or periodontal ligament stem cells, and as a direct pulp-capping material to protect exposed dental pulp from infections [58, 60].

## 2.5 Another material DPC

Eugenol Zinc Oxide (ZOE): It has been mentioned as another material for dental pulp capping, possessing bactericidal properties similar to those of CH cements and calcium silicate [10]. However, the release of eugenol from this material is highly toxic to cells [16]. A study revealed that coating dental pulp with ZOE did not result in pulp healing but rather in chronic inflammation and absence of dentin bridge formation after 12 weeks [10]. Consequently, ZOE is not recommended for dental pulp coating [10, 11].

Glass Ionomer (GI) and Resin-Modified Glass Ionomer (RMGI): While CH and calcium silicate cements are alkaline in nature, GI, RMGI cements retain their initial acidity at a low pH for an extended period, which could have an adverse impact on pulp tissue [11]. Compared to CH and GI/RMGI, CH has been shown to significantly promote pulp healing, while GI/RMGI resulted in chronic inflammation and absence of dentin bridge formation after 10 months. Therefore, GI/RMGI should not be used for dental pulp coating [9].

### *2.5.1 Bioactive glass*

Bioactive glass (BG) is a novel material that has gained significant prominence in regenerative dentistry due to its unique properties. Composed primarily of silica, calcium, and phosphorus, BG stimulates beneficial cellular responses, promoting the formation of hydroxyapatite and facilitating tissue regeneration. Its capacity to release ions and its intrinsic bioactivity make it a promising candidate for various dental applications [38, 62].

*Clinical applications of bioactive glass:*

1. Direct pulp capping: BG is utilized to promote the formation of reparative dentin and safeguard pulp vitality. It fosters the creation of a barrier between the pulp and the restorative material. BG reduces the need for pulp extirpation.

2. Repair of bone defects: BG is employed in osseous regeneration surgeries to repair bone defects, including those associated with implant dentistry. Research has demonstrated the efficacy of BG in promoting the formation of new bone tissue and integration with surrounding dental structures. BG increases the success rate of dental implants [62].

3. Regenerative endodontics: BG has shown potential in stimulating the regeneration of the dentin-pulp complex. Studies have explored its application in pulpotomies and pulpectomies, highlighting its ability to promote the formation of dentin-pulp tissue. BG offers a more conservative alternative to tooth extraction [62].

*Considerations regarding the use of adhesive materials:*

While resin adhesive materials have been recommended for their bonding ability [38]. However, despite their similarity to GI and RMGI in terms of their acidic nature and lack of bactericidal properties, adhesive resins have been found to have unsatisfactory results in terms of pulp healing and dentin bridging compared to CH [63–65]. Interestingly, studies have shown that directly coating the pulp with non-acidic adhesive resin or resin composite tends to elicit a better pulp response compared to the use of acidic primers or adhesives. Therefore, it is advisable to avoid the use of dental adhesive in DPC [9, 11].

While adhesive resin has shown promising results in experimental models during the early stages after DPC, its use in humans has revealed a lack of biocompatibility and consistent formation of reparative dentin [66].

## 3. Clinical protocol for direct pulp capping

### 3.1 Diagnosis

Implementation of DPC treatment is recommended and is performed after a comprehensive diagnosis. To accurately determine the extent of caries and fractures in the affected tooth, intraoral radiographs should be obtained. Patient history and reports, radiographic evidence, clinical evaluation, and sensitivity testing should be considered before treatment decisions are made. Once the clinical evaluation is completed and pulp exposure is confirmed, the initial pulp diagnosis can be confirmed [61].

### 3.2 Caries removal

In situations where there are cases of pulp exposure, it is of utmost importance to completely remove the caries to eradicate the infected tissues [61]. When managing deep caries lesions, it is necessary to remove demineralized enamel and infected dentin. If infected tissue is left behind, chronic inflammatory cells have been observed to infiltrate and subclinical pulp inflammation can compromise pulp vitality [25]. The use of caries detectors can be beneficial during the caries removal process, especially when working in close proximity to the pulp cavity [67, 68].

### 3.3 Use of hemostatic agent

The use of a hemostatic agent is advised in order to effectively control bleeding arising from the exposed pulp. A variety of hemostatic solutions and techniques are recommended to achieve this goal. These include, among others, sodium hypochlorite (NaOCl), chlorhexidine, hydrogen peroxide, ferric sulfate, and other similar options. Among these alternatives, the most efficient hemostatic solution for direct pulp exposure in the dental field is 2.5% NaOCl [69]. This particular solution serves as an antimicrobial agent that not only facilitates hemostasis but also disinfects the dentin-pulp interface, eradicates biofilm, chemically removes blood clots and fibrin, as well as removes dentin chips and damaged cells from the mechanically exposed site [31]. To achieve hemostasis in the exposed pulp, two main approaches have been proposed: direct passive irrigation or the use of NaOCl-soaked cotton pellets [70]. Despite the availability of multiple hemostatic options, NaOCl can be administered directly to the pulp tissue at different concentrations without compromising the integrity of the pulp itself [71]. It is of utmost importance to control bleeding prior to application of an appropriate biomaterial, as this facilitates clinical assessment of inflammation levels and identification of potential necrotic tissue.

### 3.4 Use of biomaterials

The use of biomaterials plays an important role in the successful treatment of direct pulp capping DPC. The use of calcium silicate-based materials in DPC procedures has become increasingly popular in recent years, as demonstrated by numerous studies [17, 32, 34, 72–74]. These materials have consistently demonstrated their clinical effectiveness, with MTA being one of the most widely used and investigated biomaterials in DPC [11, 73, 75]. Furthermore, compared to CH-based materials, calcium silicate-based materials have been shown to create higher quality mineralized tissue barriers and consistent mineralized tissue formation and long-term preservation of pulp vitality [76].

### 3.5 Final restoration

Final restoration of the tooth represents a fundamental phase in DPC procedures. A higher level of success is observed when teeth undergo DPC treatment using calcium silicate-based cements and are restored quickly [11, 41]. Immediate restoration confers numerous benefits, such as prevention of microleakage, protection of the biomaterial layer, mitigation of postoperative sensitivity, and improved thermal conductivity.

The results of pulpal complex regeneration (PCR) vary according to the type of lesion, the biomaterial used, the application technique, and the clinical conditions of the patient [76].

## 4. Factors affecting the results of PCR

1. Type of lesion: The severity of the pulp lesion is a crucial factor affecting the results of PCR. Mild lesions are more likely to respond positively to PCR compared to severe lesions.

2. Biomaterial used: The type of biomaterial used can also affect the results of PCR. Biomaterials that promote dentin and blood vessel formation are more likely to result in complete regeneration.

3. Application technique: The technique used to apply the biomaterial may influence the PCR results. Techniques that ensure biomaterial stability are more likely to lead to successful regeneration.

4. Clinical conditions of the patient: Patient clinical conditions, including age, general health and oral hygiene, can also affect PCR results. Young, healthy patients with good oral hygiene are more likely to respond positively to PCR [13].

## 5. Types of PCR results

1. Complete regeneration: Ideal outcome of CRP characterized by the formation of new dental pulp, including odontoblasts, dentin, and blood vessels.

2. Partial repair: Less favorable PCR outcome characterized by the formation of new dental pulp but lacking odontoblasts or blood vessels.

3. Failure: The least favorable outcome of PCR characterized by the absence of dental pulp regeneration or repair [13].

## 6. Conclusions

Dentin-pulp complex regeneration (DPCR) research is progressing rapidly. New biomaterials, techniques, and cell therapies could make DPCR a viable option for all patients in the future. DPCR is an area of research in dentistry with great potential to improve the preservation of natural teeth. New biomaterials, techniques and cell therapies are being developed that could improve regeneration outcomes. Advances in DPCR could allow dentists to preserve natural teeth in cases where extraction would have been previously indicated. This has the potential to improve patients' quality of life and decrease the costs associated with medical care. However, there are still challenges that must be overcome before DPCR becomes a viable option for all patients. These challenges include:

- The need to develop more biocompatible, bioactive, and biodegradable biomaterials.
- The need to develop more precise and efficient techniques for the application of biomaterials.
- The need to better understand the regeneration mechanisms of the dentin-pulp complex.

Traditionally, pulp inflammation has been considered only as an undesirable side effect. However, recent research indicates that it actually plays a crucial role in the pulp healing process as it leads to cell multiplication, facilitates pulp cell attachment and stimulates the proliferation of various cell types that transform into odontoblast-like cells, thus promoting the development of mineralized tissue at the site of exposure. Although calcium hydroxide has been extensively studied as a biomaterial with positive clinical results, calcium silicate-based materials currently demonstrate the highest efficacy among biomaterials used in DPCR. In addition, MTA and Biodentine have shown superior clinical results compared to other materials used in DPCR.

## Thanks

We would like to thank the Universidad Católica de Cuenca for their support in the execution of this Book Chapter, as it stems from a research project entitled PERFIL EPIDEMIOLOGICO BUCAL DE LA PROVINCIA DEL CAÑAR from the 5th call with Code PICV18-31.

## Author details

Cristian Danilo Urgiles Urgiles, Cristina Estefania Urgiles Esquivel*,
Maria Isabel Bravo, Fernanda Gonzalez and Daniela San Martin
Universidad Católica de Cuenca campus Azogues, Cañar, Ecuador

*Address all correspondence to: curgilesu@ucacue.edu.ec

## References

[1] Christie B, Musri N, Djustiana N, et al. Based materials on human advances and challenges in regenerative dentistry: A systematic review of calcium phosphate and silicatedental pulp stem cells. Materials Today Biology. 2023:1-11. Epub ahead of print 2023. DOI: 10.1016/j.mtbio.2023.100815

[2] Li B, Chen X, Jin Y. Tooth and Dental Pulp Regeneration. Elsevier Inc; 2018. Epub ahead of print 2018. DOI: 10.1016/B978-0-12-811920-4.00015-X

[3] Song M, Yu B, Kim S, et al. Clinical and molecular perspectives of reparative dentin formation: Lessons learned from pulp-capping materials and the emerging roles of calcium. Dental Clinics of North America. 2017;**61**:93-110

[4] Hou X, Zhang L, Zhou Z, et al. Calcium phosphate-based biomaterials for bone repair. Journal of Functional Biomaterials. 2022:1-39. Epub ahead of print 2022. DOI: 10.3390/jfb13040187

[5] Lin LM, Kahler B. A review of regenerative endodontics: Current protocols and future directions Rejeneratif Endodonti Üzerine Bir Derleme: Güncel Protokoller Ve Geleceğe Yönelik Öneriler. Journal of Istanbul University Faculty of Dentistry. 2017;**51**:41-51

[6] Koubi G, Colon P, Franquin JC, et al. Clinical evaluation of the performance and safety of a new dentine substitute, biodentine, in the restoration of posterior teeth - a prospective study. Clinical Oral Investigations. 2013;**17**:243-249

[7] Palczewska-komsa MP, Nowicka A. The influence of new bioactive materials on pulp – Dentin complex regeneration in the assessment of cone bone computed tomography (CBCT) and computed micro-tomography (Micro-CT) from a present and future perspective – A systematic review. Journal of Clinical Medicine. 30 May 2022;**11**(11):3091. DOI: 10.3390/jcm11113091. PMID: 35683478; PMCID: PMC9181092

[8] Bds ASA, Bds KMB, Bds MAA. The radiographic outcomes of direct pulp-capping procedures performed by dental students. Journal of the American Dental Association (1939). 2006;**137**:1699-1705

[9] Farges J, Alliot-licht B, Renard E, et al. Dental pulp defence and repair mechanisms in dental caries. Mediators of Inflammation. 2015;**2015**:230251. DOI: 10.1155/2015/230251. Epub 2015 Oct 11. PMID: 26538821; PMCID: PMC4619960

[10] Hilton TJ. Keys to clinical success with pulp capping: A review of the literature. Operative Dentistry. 2009;**34**:615-625

[11] Mente J, Hufnagel S, Leo M, et al. Treatment outcome of mineral trioxide aggregate or calcium hydroxide direct pulp capping: Long-term results. Journal of Endodontia. 2014;**40**:1746-1751

[12] Asgary S, Ahmadyar M. Vital pulp therapy using calcium-enriched mixture: An evidence-based review. Journal of Conservative Dentistry. 2013;**16**:92-98

[13] Islam R, Islam MRR, Tanaka T, et al. Direct pulp capping procedures – Evidence and practice. Japan Dental Science Review. 2023;**59**:48-61

[14] Barthel CR, Levin LG, Reisner HM, Trope M. TNF-alpha release in monocytes after exposure to calcium hydroxide treated Escherichia coli LPS. International Endodontic Journal. May

1997;**30**(3):155-159. DOI: 10.1046/j.1365-2591.1997.00066.x. PMID: 9477798

[15] Cao Y, Song M, Kim E, et al. Pulp-dentin regeneration: Current state and future prospects. Journal of Dental Research. 2015;**94**:1544-1551

[16] Ba-Hattab R, Al-Jamie M, Aldreib H, Alessa L, Alonazi M. Calcium hydroxide in endodontics: An overview. Open Journal of Stomatology. Jan 2016;**06**(12):274-289. DOI: 10.4236/ojst.2016.612033

[17] Toida Y, Kawano S, Islam R, Jiale F, Chowdhury AA, Hoshika S, et al. Pulpal response to mineral trioxide aggregate containing phosphorylated pullulan-based capping material. Dental Materials Journal. 1 Feb 2022;**41**(1):126-133. DOI: 10.4012/dmj.2021-153. Epub 2021 Oct 1. PMID: 34602588

[18] Dutta A, Saunders WP. Calcium silicate materials in endodontics. Dental Update. 2014;**41**:708-722

[19] Poggio C, Arciola CR, Beltrami R, Monaco A, Dagna A, Lombardini M, et al. Cytocompatibility and antibacterial properties of capping materials. ScientificWorldJournal. 2014;**2014**:181945. DOI: 10.1155/2014/181945. Epub 2014 May 18. PMID: 24959601; PMCID: PMC4052471

[20] Matsuura T, Ziauddin SM, Kawata-Matsuura VKS, Sugimoto K, Yamada S, Yoshimura A. Long-term clinical and radiographic evaluation of the effectiveness of direct pulp capping materials: A meta-analysis. Dental Materials Journal. 31 Jan 2021;**40**(1):1-7. DOI: 10.4012/dmj.2020-043. Epub 2020 Oct 1. PMID: 32999260

[21] Horsted P, Sandergaard B, Thylstrup A, El Attar K, Fejerskov O. A retrospective study of direct pulp capping with calcium hydroxide compounds. Endodontics and Dental Traumatology. Feb 1985;**1**(1):29-34. DOI: 10.1111/j.1600-9657.1985.tb00555.x. PMID: 3858095

[22] Arandi NZ, Rabi T. TheraCal LC: From biochemical and bioactive properties to clinical applications. International Journal of Dentistry. 26 Mar 2018;**2018**:3484653. DOI: 10.1155/2018/3484653. PMID: 29785184; PMCID: PMC5892295

[23] Camilleri J. Characterization of hydration products of mineral trioxide aggregate. International Endodontic Journal. 2008;**41**:408-417

[24] da Rosa WLO, Cocco AR, Silva TM d., et al. Current trends and future perspectives of dental pulp capping materials: A systematic review. Journal of Biomedical Materials Research – Part B Applied Biomaterials 2018;106:1358-1368

[25] Smith AJ. Pulpal responses to caries and dental repair. Caries Research. Jul-Aug 2002;**36**(4):223-232. DOI: 10.1159/000063930. PMID: 12218270

[26] Lipski M, Nowicka A, Kot K, et al. Factors affecting the outcomes of direct pulp capping using biodentine. Clinical Oral Investigations. 2018;**22**:2021-2029

[27] Okiji T, Yoshiba K. Reparative dentinogenesis induced by mineral trioxide aggregate: A review from the biological and physicochemical points of view. International Journal of Dentistry. 2009;**2009**:464280. DOI: 10.1155/2009/464280. Epub 2009 Dec 28. PMID: 20339574; PMCID: PMC2837314

[28] Nair PN, Duncan HF, Pitt Ford TR, Luder HU. Histological, ultrastructural and quantitative investigations on the

response of healthy human pulps to experimental capping with mineral trioxide aggregate: A randomized controlled trial. International Endodontic Journal. May 2009;**42**(5):422-444. DOI: 10.1111/j.1365-2591.2009.01558.x. PMID: 19356180

[29] Bogen G, Kim JS, Bakland LK. Direct pulp capping with mineral trioxide aggregate: An observational study. Journal of the American Dental Association (1939). 2008;**139**:305-315

[30] Kuratate M, Yoshiba K, Shigetani Y, Yoshiba N, Ohshima H, Okiji T. Immunohistochemical analysis of nestin, osteopontin, and proliferating cells in the reparative process of exposed dental pulp capped with mineral trioxide aggregate. Journal of Endodontics. Aug 2008;**34**(8):970-974. DOI: 10.1016/j.joen.2008.03.021. Epub 2008 Jun 20. PMID: 18634929

[31] AAE position statement on vital pulp therapy. Journal of Endodontics. Sep 2021;**47**(9):1340-1344. DOI: 10.1016/j.joen.2021.07.015. Epub 2021 Aug 3. PMID: 34352305

[32] Komabayashi T, Zhu Q, Eberhart R, Imai Y. Current status of direct pulp-capping materials for permanent teeth current status of direct pulp-capping materials for permanent teeth. Dental Materials Journal. 2016;**35**(1):1-12. DOI: 10.4012/dmj.2015-013. PMID: 26830819

[33] Silva GAB, Gava E, Lanza LD, et al. Subclinical failures of direct pulp capping of human teeth by using a dentin bonding system. Journal of Endodontia. 2013;**39**:182-189

[34] Nie E, Yu J, Jiang R, et al. Effectiveness of direct pulp capping bioactive materials in dentin regeneration: A systematic review. Materials (Basel). 11 Nov 2021;**14**(22):6811. DOI: 10.3390/ma14226811. PMID: 34832214; PMCID: PMC8621741

[35] Tselnik M, Baumgartner JC, Marshall JG. Bacterial leakage with mineral trioxide aggregate or a resin-modified glass ionomer used as a coronal barrier. Journal of Endodontics. Nov 2004;**30**(11):782-784. DOI: 10.1097/00004770-200411000-00008. PMID: 15505510

[36] Jang Y, Song M, Yoo IS, Song Y, Roh BD, Kim E. A randomized controlled study of the use of ProRoot mineral trioxide aggregate and endocem as direct pulp capping materials: 3-month versus 1-year outcomes. Journal of Endodontics. Aug 2015;**41**(8):1201-1206. DOI: 10.1016/j.joen.2015.03.015. Epub 2015 Apr 29. PMID: 25933707

[37] Baskaran S, Ahamed AS, Narayana SS. Original article a randomized controlled study of the use of mineral trioxide aggregate angelus (white) and biodentine as pulp capping materials. Endodontology. Jan 2018;**30**(1):69-75. DOI: 10.4103/endo.endo_54_17

[38] Chen L, Suh BI. Cytotoxicity and biocompatibility of resin-free and resin-modified direct pulp capping materials: A state-of-the-art review. Dental Materials Journal. 2017;**36**:1-7

[39] Wang C, Yi Z, Tian L, et al. Development of a novel biodegradable and anti-bacterial polyurethane coating for biomedical magnesium rods. Materials Science & Engineering C. 2019;**99**:344-356

[40] Neves ADA, Coutinho E, De MJ, et al. Caries-removal effectiveness and minimal-invasiveness potential of caries-excavation techniques : A micro-CT investigation. Journal of Dentistry. 2011;**39**:154-162

[41] About I. Recent trends in tricalcium silicates for vital pulp therapy

[42] Arandi NZ, Thabet M. Minimal intervention in dentistry: A literature review on biodentine as a bioactive pulp capping material. Biomedical Research International. 3 Apr 2021;**2021**:5569313. DOI: 10.1155/2021/5569313. PMID: 33884264; PMCID: PMC8041541

[43] Camilleri J. Investigation of the hydration and bioactivity of radiopaci fi ed tricalcium silicate cement. Biodentine and MTA Angelus. 2013;**9**:580-593

[44] Grech L, Mallia B, Camilleri J. Investigation of the physical properties of tricalcium silicate cement-based root-end filling materials. Dental Materials. 2012;**29**:e20-e28

[45] Kaur M, Singh H, Dhillon JS, Batra M, Saini M. MTA versus biodentine: Review of literature with a comparative analysis. Journal of Clinical and Diagnostic Research. Aug 2017;**11**(8):ZG01-ZG05. DOI: 10.7860/JCDR/2017/25840.10374. Epub 2017 Aug 1. PMID: 28969295; PMCID: PMC5620936

[46] Al-Sherbiny IM, Farid MH, Abu-Seida AM, et al. Chemico-physical and mechanical evaluation of three calcium silicate-based pulp capping materials. Saudi Dental Journal. 2021;**33**:207-214

[47] Gandolfi MG, Siboni F, Botero T, et al. Calcium silicate and calcium hydroxide materials for pulp capping: Biointeractivity, porosity, solubility and bioactivity of current formulations. Journal of Applied Biomaterials & Functional Materials. 2015;**13**:1-18

[48] Li X, Yoshihara K, De Munck J, Cokic S, Pongprueksa P, Putzeys E, et al. Modified tricalcium silicate cement formulations with added zirconium oxide. Clinical Oral Investigations. Apr 2017;**21**(3):895-905. DOI: 10.1007/s00784-016-1843-y. Epub 2016 May 7. PMID: 27153848

[49] Natale LC, Rodrigues MC, Xavier TA, et al. Ion release and mechanical properties of calcium silicate and calcium hydroxide materials used for pulp capping. International Endodontic Journal. 2015;**48**:89-94

[50] Giraud T, Jeanneau C, Rombouts C, et al. Pulp capping materials modulate the balance between inflammation and regeneration. Dental Materials. 2019;**35**:24-35

[51] Nowicka A, Lipski M, Parafiniuk M, et al. Response of human dental pulp capped with biodentine and mineral trioxide aggregate. Journal of Endodontia. 2013;**39**:743-747

[52] Camilleri J, Laurent P, About I. Hydration of biodentine, theracal LC, and a prototype tricalcium silicate-based dentin replacement material after pulp capping in entire tooth cultures. Journal of Endodontia. 2014;**40**:1846-1854

[53] Parirokh M, Torabinejad M. Calcium silicate – Based cements. In: Torabinejad M, editor. Mineral Trioxide Aggregate: Properties and Clinical Applications, 1st ed. John Wiley & Sons, Inc.; 2014

[54] Zhu L, Yang J, Zhang J, Peng B. A comparative study of BioAggregate and ProRoot MTA on adhesion, migration, and attachment of human dental pulp cells. Journal of Endodontics. Aug 2014;**40**(8):1118-1123. DOI: 10.1016/j.joen.2013.12.028. Epub 2014 Feb 5. PMID: 25069918

[55] Inami C, Endoh C, Ichinohe H, et al. Original effect of direct pulp capping

with a novel chemically curable mineral trioxide aggregate material using tri-butylborane as a polymerization initiator. Journal of Hard Tissue Biology. 2019:383-390

[56] Gandolfi MG, Siboni F, Prati C. Chemical-physical properties of TheraCal, a novel light-curable MTA-like material for pulp capping. International Endodontic Journal. 2012;**45**:571-579

[57] Peskersoy C, Lukarcanin J, Turkun M. Efficacy of different calcium silicate materials as pulp-capping agents: Randomized clinical trial. Journal of Dental Sciences. Mar 2021;**16**(2):723-731. DOI: 10.1016/j.jds.2020.08.016. Epub 2020 Sep 17. PMID: 33854725; PMCID: PMC8025185

[58] Abbass MMS, El-Rashidy AA, Sadek KM, et al. Hydrogels and dentin–pulp complex regeneration: From the benchtop to clinical translation. Polymers (Basel). 2020;**12**:1-65

[59] Deng R, Xie Y, Chan U, et al. Biomaterials and biotechnology for periodontal tissue regeneration: Recent advances and perspectives. Journal of Dental Research, Dental Clinics, Dental Prospects. 2022;**16**:1-10

[60] Zhao L, Zhou Y, Zhang J, Liang H, Chen X, Tan H. Natural polymer-based hydrogels: From polymer to biomedical applications. Pharmaceutics. 23 Oct 2023;**15**(10):2514. DOI: 10.3390/pharmaceutics15102514. PMID: 37896274; PMCID: PMC10610124

[61] Karchoubi F, Ghotli RA, Pahlevani H, et al. Advanced industrial and engineering polymer research new insights into nanocomposite hydrogels: A review on recent advances in characteristics and applications. Advanced Industrial and Engineering Polymer Research. 2024;**7**:54-78

[62] Kunert M, Lukomska-Szymanska M. Bio-inductive materials in direct and indirect pulp capping – A review article. Materials (Basel). 2020;**7**:13. Epub ahead of print 2020. DOI: 10.3390/ma13051204

[63] Reyes-Carmona JF, Santos ARS, Figueiredo CP, et al. In vivo host interactions with mineral trioxide aggregate and calcium hydroxide: Inflammatory molecular signaling assessment. Journal of Endodontia. 2011;**37**:1225-1235

[64] Cannio M, Bellucci D, Roether JA, Boccaccini DN, Cannillo V. Bioactive glass applications: A literature review of human clinical trials. Materials (Basel). 20 Sep 2021;**14**(18):5440. DOI: 10.3390/ma14185440. PMID: 34576662; PMCID: PMC8470635

[65] Ricucci D, Siqueira JF, Rôças IN, et al. Pulp and dentine responses to selective caries excavation : A histological and histobacteriological human study. Journal of Dentistry. 2020;**100**:103430

[66] da Modena KC, Casas-Apayco LC, Atta MT, et al. Cytotoxicity and biocompatibility of direct and indirect pulp capping materials. Journal of Applied Oral Science. 2009;**17**:544-554

[67] Hosoya Y, Taguchi T, Tay FR. Evaluation of a new caries detecting dye for primary and permanent carious dentin. Journal of Dentistry. Feb 2007;**35**(2):137-143. DOI: 10.1016/j.jdent.2006.06.004. Epub 2006 Sep 1. PMID: 16945461

[68] Souza RA, Gomes SC, Dantas Jda C, Silva-Sousa YT, Pécora JD. Importance of the diagnosis in the pulpotomy of immature permanent teeth. Brazilian Dental Journal. 2007;**18**(3):244-247. DOI: 10.1590/s0103-64402007000300013. PMID: 18176718

[69] Ballal NV, Duncan HF, Rai N, et al. Sodium hypochlorite reduces postoperative discomfort and painful early failure after carious exposure and direct pulp capping – Initial findings of a randomized controlled trial. Journal of Clinical Medicine. 28 Jul 2020;**9**(8):2408. DOI: 10.3390/jcm9082408. PMID: 32731401; NPMCID: PMC7464668

[70] Cho S, Seo D, Lee S. Prognostic factors for clinical outcomes according to time after direct pulp capping. Journal of Endodontia. 2013;**39**:327-331

[71] Mds KS, Mds JD, Mds ST, et al. Success of direct pulp capping using mineral trioxide aggregate and calcium hydroxide in mature permanent molars with pulps exposed during carious tissue removal : 1-year follow-up. Journal of Endodontia. 2019;**45**:840-847

[72] Demetrescu I. The effect of calcium-silicate cements on reparative dentinogenesis following direct pulp capping on animal models molecules. 6 May 2021;**26**(9):2725. DOI: 10.3390/molecules26092725. PMID: 34066444; PMCID: PMC8125639

[73] Çalışkan MK, Güneri P. Prognostic factors in direct pulp capping with mineral trioxide aggregate or calcium hydroxide: 2- to 6-year follow-up. Clinical Oral Investigations. Jan 2017;**21**(1):357-367. DOI: 10.1007/s00784-016-1798-z. Epub 2016 Apr 4. PMID: 27041110

[74] Dammaschke T, Leidinger J, Schäfer E. Long-term evaluation of direct pulp capping--treatment outcomes over an average period of 6.1 years. Clinical Oral Investigations. Oct 2010;**14**(5):559-567. DOI: 10.1007/s00784-009-0326-9. Epub 2009 Aug 15. PMID: 19685086

[75] Hilton TJ, Ferracane JL, Mancl L; Northwest Practice-based Research Collaborative in Evidence-based Dentistry (NWP). Comparison of CaOH with MTA for direct pulp capping: A PBRN randomized clinical trial. Journal of Dental Research. Jul 2013;**92**(7 Suppl):16S-22S. DOI: 10.1177/0022034513484336. Epub 2013 May 20. PMID: 23690353; PMCID: PMC3706175

[76] McComb D. Caries-detector dyes--how accurate and useful are they? Journal of the Canadian Dental Association. Apr 2000;**66**(4):195-198. PMID: 10789171